ACID REFLUX FORMULA

Overcome Acid Reflux Permanently

Fundamentals of Healing

DREW NIEMEYER

Reader's Bonus

If you want some immediate relief from acid reflux pain while you start to put the *Acid Reflux Formula* into action, download my full guide to relieving symptoms here: **https://acidrefluxformula.com/book-bonus**

Remember to log back into Amazon and leave a review for this book. This will help other readers to find this information more easily.

Good luck with your progress in solving your reflux dilemmas. Please stay in contact with me using the information on the last page, and write to me about your questions, your dilemmas and your successes!

Disclaimer

This book contains the opinions and ideas of its author, and is to be used for informational purposes only. It is sold with the understanding that the author and publisher are not engaged in rendering medical, health, or any other kind of personal professional services in the book. The author and publisher specifically disclaim all responsibility for any liability, loss, or risk — personal or otherwise — that is incurred as a consequence, directly or indirectly, of the use and application of any of the contents of this book. A health-care professional should be consulted regarding your specific medical situation. Any product mentioned in this book does not imply endorsement of that product by the author or publisher.

Many of the designations used by manufacturers and sellers to distinguish their products are claimed as trademarks. Where those designations appear in this book and Drew Niemeyer was aware of a trademark claim, the designations have been printed in initial capital letters.

CONTENTS

INTRODUCTION

There are many books about reflux out there that fail to reach the true causes of reflux disease. You may have read several of them. Some focus on a single cause by implementing a FODMAP diet, or by eliminating a food sensitivity, and others focus on managing the symptoms through low-acid diets and other smaller measures.

This book is about the most significant discoveries I made over the last twenty years in my quest to overcome reflux disease. I have never been content to simply manage the disease. After all, a low acid diet is not a permanent fix. A low-acid diet is, without doubt, the best way to manage the symptoms, but the underlying disease is still there. My research, instead, is more focused on discovering the underlying causes of reflux disease and the ways to fix them.

Where is the Cure?

All the information we need to overcome reflux disease is already available to the general public. You might be surprised to hear this, and you might have tried many different strategies to overcome the pain already, without success. One problem is that the answers are hidden amongst conflicting information. Another problem is that no one follows the correct sequence of steps to ensure that reflux disease is cured.

The sequence of steps is important. This book will walk you through the difficulties of reversing reflux disease. You cannot simply open a random chapter such as gut health and expect that you can focus on that one method. Every chapter of this book is dependent on the chapters that come before it. If you have not followed the sequence of steps correctly, you are more likely to fail in your attempts to fix the problem. This includes when and how to give up PPI medication, or when to start thinking about gut health.

This book is part 1 in a three-part series on the real causes of reflux disease. Although I would like to have contained everything in one single book, I felt that the volume of material would make some people give up before they ever started. Despite the length of the book(s), remember that this is just a 'mud-map' for your journey to health. It is a very brief explanation of all the points that you need to know and is not a comprehensive treatise on the subjects. Every chapter tackles a subject that could easily expand to become a book of its own.

For the sake of offering you a read that is short and manageable, I have tried to include only the most relevant information. The purpose is to provide a comprehensive overview of the topic that can provide some direction for your own research, and solid information for discussion with your doctor.

Why I Wrote This Book

The pain of reflux disease is very difficult for others to understand. Not only is the pain severe, it is persistent, and no one wants to hear about our constant complaints. The pain from my own reflux was severe. Every night, throughout the entire night, I could feel it building up and by the time morning came, my throat and my sinuses, were red raw. It felt as though a severe cold had hit me during the night. My throat was swollen, my vocal chords were also swollen, and it was very difficult and painful to speak. My dentist warned me that my back teeth were also being eroded. This was my life every day.

And it is not just about the physical pain. Other people think less of you because you need to turn down invitations to celebrations, to food events and even to physical activities. For a few years I never had time for anything much other than managing my reflux symptoms. Life was exhausting. I would try to relieve the pain in the morning before work, and in the evenings, I spent the whole time preparing my special reflux-minimizing food for the next day, navigating the minefield of foods that might trigger more reflux episodes. And if I had to go out with others, I needed to prepare for that in addition to everything else that I was trying to do. That was just to manage the symptoms, and ensure the pain was minimized as much as possible.

In my desperation to escape the pain, I visited many types of doctors and experimented with many different types of foods and medicines. I tried plant-based, vegetarian, high-fibre, wholegrain, sprouted seeds and nuts, and all organic foods. I did loads of reading and tried out many different types of supplements including HCl, vitamins, minerals etc. Aside from the specialists, I saw nutritionists, naturopaths, allergists and I tried to pinpoint problems through elimination diets. I tried to improve my digestion with bitter herbs and tinctures or by using parasite cleanses.

I was someone that wanted to believe in our medicines, in natural medicines, organic and health foods, and I was let down.

But those were the worst failures of 10+ years ago. I have since found exactly the solution I was looking for and therefore I have written this book. I want to share my journey with you and help you to relieve your own pain, too.

I know how it feels. I often meet people who are convinced that no one could be experiencing pain worse than their own, but I am here to tell you that it can be overcome. You can conquer this pain, even if you think that you have tried 'everything'.

Is This Book for You?

While this book provides the knowledge to identify the causes of your reflux, you need to be aware that some people may not benefit from it as much as others do.

Firstly, this book has been formulated specially for those with LPR (Laryngopharyngeal Reflux, or silent reflux). This is the form of reflux that affected me, but if you have another form of reflux disease, I highly encourage you to read this book. The principles that I outline may still be of great value to you.

Secondly, there are sections of the community that will not benefit from everything that I have written here. This is especially the case for those who:

- have missing organs such as the LES (lower esophageal sphincter)
- have had surgery to remove organs (eg. Gallbladder)
- have had surgery on the intestines (re-section)
- have had a procedure on the stomach or LES to prevent reflux from occurring

This book may be of limited value for you if you fall into these categories. There is valuable information to be had, but you may need to follow additional guidelines that properly support your particular physical condition.

Thirdly, your particular values may not align with this book. For devoted vegans and vegetarians, this book may not be appropriate if you are determined to remain on plant-based diets. Although it may be possible to overcome reflux on a plant-based diet, I do not believe it is optimal.

Many people believe that animal products are holding back their health, and I believed the same for a long time. The results of my tests and elimination diets showed that animal products were causing many of my issues. Also, nutritional experts support plant-based diets, and plant-based diets are currently the strongest recommendations for managing reflux disease.

But I want to achieve more than merely managing the disease. Through a combination of chance and a little desperation, I found the results were better when there were less plants and more animal products. I am sure that it is possible to overcome reflux on a plant-based diet, but I believe this is the slow-lane on a very long and difficult road. Many people will never reach its destination. The chapters in this book are not written to disparage any path to healing. They simply outline the steps that worked best for me, why it worked for me, and why it also works for the majority of other people.

For anyone who is open to change, I hope that these pages will become an effective springboard from which you can launch your own research. Most people will find relief from acid reflux within the first major step in this book, but please keep reading the entire book: the goal is to keep acid reflux away for good.

In addition to this, I urge you to act quickly! The diseases that cause acid reflux tend to degrade the functionality of the body as time goes by. The information in this book becomes less effective the longer symptoms continue and damage to the body's organs becomes increasingly permanent. The best solution is to overcome the causes of reflux as soon as possible, before the reflux-causing diseases have set in for good.

Can Acid Reflux Really be Cured?

There will always be instances where reflux cannot be cured, and instances when it can. The key to understanding reflux is this: Reflux is always caused by other diseases.

If you have spent time on forums and discussions, you may have discovered that everyone with reflux also has a list of other health complaints. Deciding on whether Acid Reflux can be cured depends on how you understand the disease.

This is the basic premise of this book.

Over the years, I have noticed that reflux is always accompanied by other diseases. Taking steps to identify these diseases and to fix them is key to overcoming reflux.

So, is acid reflux curable? This depends on what underlying disease is causing your reflux, and how permanently that disease has damaged your body. If the underlying disease is curable, then I believe you will cure your reflux. Thankfully, this is the case for most people.

If your body has been permanently damaged from a disease, and this disease continues to affect your health (this can happen from autoimmune disease or from organ damage from incorrect lifestyle choices), then you may be able to manage acid reflux by managing the underlying disease. Many people in this situation continue to improve slowly over time, but it is difficult to know how far that improvement will go.

How to Optimize Your Progress

The information contained in the coming chapters is no replacement for your relationship with a team of medical professionals.

This book is not about changing your allegiance, but more about dissemination of valuable material. Essentially, it is unfair to hold back on information when other people could be using it for their own benefit, no matter how anecdotal it may seem. Experience and research are important tools in the search for answers to our health concerns, and it is my own experiences and research that you will find written here.

Many people regard overcoming disease naturally as being hippie, trendy or radical. This is not my intention. The fact is that even conventional medicine has no drug that cures or manages reflux safely. The only option we have for curing reflux is via natural methods. And the guidance of a good doctor is absolutely necessary while you are travelling this path.

With this information in hand, you must find a doctor that can collaborate in your efforts to cure your reflux. This book does not offer any advice to your specific circumstances and I hope that the information in this book can be a valuable resource in this journey.

I often hear people tearing down the medical establishment because they feel that they have been ignored and left out to dry. It is difficult to confirm these types of claims, but most medical professionals really are there to provide the greatest help that they can.

They are real people that feel a great sense of pride in obtaining positive outcomes. But they do have to work within a system.

The medical industry is not perfect. There are many barriers in the way for everyone. There are barriers holding doctors back from what they want to achieve and there are barriers in front of the patients that are looking for answers. Just knowing that there are barriers can help you to find your place within the system so that you can get the help that you need.

Firstly, information from new research takes almost 20 years to filter down to medical practice for the general public. This is a very long time that people are left without the answers that they are looking for. If you want to be up to date with the latest findings, then it is good to place yourself in the organizations that are likely to have access to this. These days, communication from researchers is excellent, and there are also many lay people that are committed to learning about new developments and broadcasting them to the world. Make sure you connect with those in the know and make yourself as informed as you can be. This will help you when discussing with doctors.

Secondly, specialists tend to limit their study to specific parts of the body, and they don't cross the boundaries to other parts of the body. This is simply the way the system trains specialists and sets them up for medical practice. This can be a problem in identifying cause and effect in diseases that involve multiple systems in the body. There are many specialists that do not collaborate deeply with other specialists, so it may be up to you to bring any relevant information to the table. Most specialists like to feel that they are informed so it may be worth asking their opinion on any connections that you have discovered in your own research.

Thirdly, any doctor, in general, must abide by conventional guidelines, or risk having their medical licenses revoked. This protects people from quackery and dangerous advice, but it also makes many doctors afraid to mention information that could be the answer to your prayers. Within the last 10 years, many lawsuits have been filed against doctors that have given excellent advice, but it was advice that their peers did not agree with or thought was unconventional. Thankfully, each of the doctors won their cases because their advice was overwhelmingly supported by the medical literature. They kept their careers, probably owing to the skill of their lawyers. But this is the danger that any doctor faces. Keep this in mind when you speak with them. They must be vigilant about staying within the boundaries that medical authorities have set.

Fourthly, general practitioners are extremely busy people. They must deal with every disease in the book – not just yours. It is impossible for a single person to understand everything in detail and that is why we have specialists. They often rely on summaries of diseases and treatments from publications for their ongoing education, usually supplied by pharmaceutical companies. Being well informed about your own condition can also be a great source of education for a practitioner.

Despite all these limitations, many doctors have found ways to help their patients without upsetting their peers. It is important to find a doctor that is open-minded and can respect your desire to research your own topic and approach them for their professional opinions on those research items. I have been lucky to find a doctor that is willing to listen to my thoughts, reasonings and to work with me in the way that I feel comfortable, and I know that you can find a doctor like this, too.

And the fifth barrier to your health, sadly, is often the pharmaceutical companies. They are in the businesses of providing products that can improve health, or fight disease and save lives where no other options exist, but they are not a charity. If there is no money involved, then the business will fold, so just like any business. They conduct themselves like businesses, they employ strategies to market their products and to make more sales, whether you need the products or not. They do play a vital role in medicine but taking pharmaceutical products unnecessarily may be making you sicker, as we will see in the following pages. There is no pharmaceutical drug that cures acid reflux because acid reflux can be cured naturally. And because of the nature of acid reflux, we are unlikely to see a cure for this disease for a very long time, if ever at all.

In the end, it is up to you to be informed, and to bring your information to doctors that are open-minded to work with you through this.

I hope that the ideas in this book can help you overcome all these barriers. The information is new, it is based on research, it has worked for other people and it is something that you can take to your doctor for discussion. The information in this book provides solutions that will cost you extraordinarily little, because acid reflux can be overcome naturally.

And Just One More Thing...

Before you continue to chapter one, I want to leave you with something to do. I want you to succeed in your efforts to overcome this disease. If you want to make the most of this book, and the suggestions that are included throughout the chapters, you would do well to include two lifestyle changes, if you are not doing them already.

One change is exercise. I know that the 'talk' about exercise can be like switching on the broken record. I totally get it. But think about doing something simple and easy. Just go walking. Put aside some time daily. Even twice daily if it's easy exercise. This is not about weight loss, but a lot of the benefits of exercise are implied throughout the pages of this book.

And the other change is to relax. And this includes getting proper sleep. Make sure you are not living in a stressful and toxic environment, and that you are as relaxed as you can be for most of your day. The fact is that stress may be causing your reflux, and if this is the case, the only solution is to remove the cause. However, if you find it difficult to relax and you want some tools that can increase your ability to relax, then the answers are in the book you are holding!

I'm not going elaborate on exercise and relaxation here because they will be big topics in book three. However, I mention them here because you can take care of these changes straight away, they can make an enormous impact to your progress, and why wait until book three to start on something that you can do right now?

Yours Sincerely,

Drew Niemeyer
Founder of *Acid Reflux Formula*

CHAPTER 1

IS WEIGHT LOSS REALLY THE ANSWER?

Doctors have little to offer patients when it comes to reflux disease. This is not to disparage them in any way. It is just that they know that there is no cure for reflux disease. The best they can do is to offer some lifestyle advice, perhaps some dietary advice, and prescribe some medications that can ease the pain.

Some of the doctors' visits I have heard about are very funny, especially the stories from skinny people. A new patient with a BMI of 21 (very thin) can visit a doctor with a complaint about reflux and be met with the words "You need to lose weight". It is as if the doctor has not even looked at the patient sitting in the room.

Although these types of situations seem incredulous, there is more truth to it than you might think. Take it from me, a tall skinny guy that has never wavered from a weight of 72kg. I knew that there was fat, and not weight, that was contributing to my reflux. Are you confused yet? Let's take a look at how this works.

How Much Does Your Weight Contribute to Reflux?

The reason that fat contributes to reflux disease, they say, is that excess fat puts pressure on your internal organs, including your stomach, and pushes the stomach contents upward into your esophagus.

Personally, I would take this reasoning with a grain of salt. I am sure that there is truth behind putting pressure on your organs, but I believe it is a small detail in the larger scheme of things. In my opinion, there is much more to the story. Excess weight is a visible sign of some other, much more serious, cause of reflux disease.

Almost every person diagnosed with acid reflux has heard these words "You have to lose weight".

Whether you are skinny or plus sized, as strange as it may sound, weight loss is something that you need to think about. This is because everybody has a particular fat capacity. Once you go over this capacity, then that is when things start to go wrong.

Some plus sized people can remain very big, and be absolutely fine because they have not yet reached their capacity. And skinny people can put on just a tiny amount of weight and already be over capacity.

How does this work? I found the whole story to be incredibly intriguing.

The Reflux/Body-Fat Connection

The link between acid reflux disease and body-fat was a mystery to me until I read some research that connected BMI with acid reflux.

The researchers were baffled by this very same question. Why do some very overweight people never develop disease, while other much thinner people are hit by the disease severely? Is body-weight not a real factor?

The data in the research was confusing. It did not matter if people had a BMI of 24 or 29 or 36. There seemed to be no pattern to the numbers.

But soon, researchers noticed something odd. The researchers could observe participants over a long period of time, so it gave them the opportunity to see the participants gain and lose weight as time passed. They watched disease develop and then disappear.

And then an idea struck. Instead of looking at all the people as one big average number, they began to study what happened to individuals as they constantly changed weight.

It became clear that a single person would develop disease after crossing above a particular weight threshold. And that same person would overcome the disease by losing those extra kilos, to bring their weight back underneath that threshold.

So, one person with a BMI of 20 would develop symptoms once their weight reached a BMI of 24. And once they took off those extra kilos they had gained, the symptoms disappeared also. Another person who already had a BMI of 32 was perfectly fine until their weight climbed to a BMI of 36. At this point they became sick. After bringing their weight back to a BMI of 34, everything went back to normal.

It was clear from his research that he could not just pick one number that would apply to everyone. At a BMI of 30, some people would develop disease and other people would not.

But what he did find, is that everyone has their own personal threshold - their ability to store fat in safe places. That is, to store fat under the skin. After this subcutaneous (skin) storage is filled, then other places need to be found where fat can be stored.

It is a little bit like people who own, and hoard, too many possessions. They need to have places inside their houses that allow them to store their things neatly and safely, without getting in the way of day-to-day activities. As belongings accumulate, the cupboard space in the house will normally get filled up first, and then any extra storage spaces. That is where the usual storage space is.

How much storage space is there in a house? That depends on the house. Some houses have a lot of storage space and others have very little. Most apartments have even less space available for storage than houses on a block of land.

Whatever the storage space capacity is, it gets filled up, and any further items need to be put in places that are not made for storage - skillfully placed or stacked on table edges or they begin taking up space in a spare room. As more and more items accumulate, it takes up more and more of the living space in the house until there are only little paths left to navigate from room to room.

The same concept happens in your body. Fat storage happens under the skin. How much can you store under the skin? That depends on you. Some people like me cannot store much under the skin, but other people can store a lot.

After this space is filled, other places need to be found. Fat will be supplied to all tissues of the body, expanding the belly, being deposited around the organs, and inside the organs. It even makes its way around and inside the cells of the organs.

Having so much fat in the wrong places makes it difficult for the body's organs to work properly. The liver gets blocked up. It stops producing particles that it needs to produce. The pancreas stops producing insulin. In general, excess fat impedes organ function.

With everything blocked up, they cannot function anymore, and they begin to also develop inflammation.

Think about fatty liver disease - you have probably heard of this - where fat is piling up inside the liver, blocking up the ducts, and preventing it from functioning properly. And visceral fat accumulating in and around the pancreas. It tends to block up the cells that create the hormones we need.

That is why we hear news of scientists that discover a 3-day fast adds functionality to the pancreas. Great news for diabetics, but the reason for the sudden "restarting" of the pancreas is that the hormone-producing cells have been uncovered and are beginning to function properly once again.

The only course of action is to treat your body as your temple. Clean out the house! Clear the clutter and regain your health.

There is much more to the story of fat than simply blocking up the organs. By now you might realize that some people can safely and happily store more fat than other people. But once that limit is reached, then that person is beginning a state of inflammation.

How Excess Fat Causes Disease

Obesity is often referred to as a chronic state of inflammation. This means that if you are over your personal fat threshold, then your body begins to send out distress signals that start the process of inflammation.

Fat cells under the skin are made for storing fat. They just keep taking in fat until they reach their limit. After that, they deal with the situation in one of 2 ways. They can either just stop taking in more fat, or they can split to form new fat cells so that the process of fat storage can continue.

Which type of cells do you have? The fat from the cells that keep dividing is quite wobbly. Many people don't like the appearance of this type of fat because all the body parts tend to wobble around. But this is the safest kind of fat.

These types of fat cells do not get stressed and overfilled, and they help to make your personal fat capacity increase. This is what helps to keep all sorts of weight-related diseases away.

On the other hand, fat that appears quite solid may be a sign of over-full fat cells. If the fat on your body is like this, then your personal fat threshold is likely reached. Your fat cells have grown too large, and they have become tight. You are now probably depositing fat into all the wrong places.

In addition to this, fat cells that are over-full start sending out stress signals that start a cascade of inflammatory responses by the body.

When fat cells grow too big, inflammatory proteins called cytokines flow out of the fat cells. This action switches on inflammatory processes throughout the whole body, especially the liver and the muscles. And it doesn't stop here. Those cytokines cause many other reactions to take place, and they all have the effect of accelerating the process: more fat storage, more inflammation and more sickness.

Complications of Inflammation

When inflammation is causing a continuous spiral into sickness, this condition is known as chronic inflammation.

Chronic inflammation is the cause of many diseases such as diabetes and heart disease. It can affect the kidneys, the bones, and is connected to autoimmune disorders and even brain diseases such as dementia and Alzheimer's.

As the inflammatory processes continue, they can create a broad spectrum of diseases. See if you recognize a few of these common ones:

- Arthritis
- Asthma
- Allergies
- Crohn's, ulcerative colitis and other auto-inflammatory diseases
- Dermatitis, Eczema
- Fibromyalgia
- IBS
- Interstitial Cystitis
- Joint Pain
- Multiple Sclerosis
- Nephritis
- Sarcoidosis

Inflammation is serious and it is currently a very popular topic within the medical community. Inflammation causes insulin resistance, which leads to acid reflux. You should always be vigilant about trying to reduce inflammation as much as possible.

And the first step in that path for most people is about losing weight.

Why Do We Gain Weight?

When it comes to our food, our bodies will do one of two things. It will use it, or it will store it. It never carries out the two processes at the same time. Just one or the other.

Think of pendulum of a clock. It swings back and forth, from one extreme to the other. In the same way, our bodies need to have the time when we are burning fat, and time when we are storing fat.

The biggest cause of fat storage in our bodies (but not the only one) is a hormone called insulin. It is produced by the pancreas and is released any time that we eat food.

Insulin is a fat-storage hormone, so it is impossible for the body to burn fat while it is around. Insulin is released when blood glucose (sugar) levels are too high. While it is present, all the body's processes are geared toward storing fat, and to storing glucose, fatty acids and amino acids (amino acids are parts of proteins). Insulin is all about stocking up on what we need.

Insulin signals for the liver to build glycogen from glucose, fats (triglycerides) from glycerol and fatty acids, and proteins from amino acids. This is all for the sake of storage and growth!

When a meal is finished and has taken two or three hours to digest, the environment starts to calm down. Then the pendulum is now swinging the other way. We are moving out of fat storage mode and into fat burning mode.

Glucagon is the opposite of insulin. It is also released from the pancreas, but this happens when blood glucose levels become too low. It signals for the liver to release some glucose into the bloodstream. When there is no insulin, some other organs begin releasing hormones that start the process of using internal stores of energy. This is not essential to our discussion, but for the sake of interest, here are the main ones:

- pancreas - glucagon
- pituitary gland - growth hormone

- pituitary gland - ACTH (adrenocorticotropic hormone)
- adrenal gland - epinephrine (adrenaline)
- thyroid gland - thyroid hormone

These hormones act on the cells of the liver, the muscles and fat tissues. And if we continue to avoid food, our fat-burning state continues. This stage of the cycle is important, not only because it is about fat burning, but because it is a time when the body takes steps to repair itself.

These two states work well because insulin is all about storage and growth, and the other hormones are about fat-burning and repair. Two different states that do two important tasks.

Now that you know that insulin is released at mealtimes, what do you think would occur if we did not stop eating, or had our meals too close together? What do you think happens when we break up our 3 largest meals of the day, and instead have 6 small meals in a day?

Frequent Small Meals

Eating frequent small meals is the advice given to many patients of reflux disease, but it leads to the condition of reflux disease becoming much worse over time.

Here is what happens. You wake up and have breakfast, at perhaps 8am. From this point, you need to eat every 2 or 2.5 hours, to be able to fit in 6 meals for the day.

After each meal, blood glucose rises, insulin is released, and the body's cells take in the glucose they need. All the extra glucose that is left is stored as fat. This whole process takes a couple of hours before it is winding up and preparing to switch over to fat-burning mode. But it is too late because it is now time for the next meal.

The next meal is eaten. Glucose enters the body again in another wave, forcing the release of more insulin. The cells of your body probably don't need any more energy right now, so most of the glucose from that meal will probably get turned into fat. Some fat cells may take in some glucose to turn it into fat, but the liver will convert most of it. And then the fat gets stored. Once again, the whole process lasts for a couple of hours, and is winding up just in time for the next meal.

The lack of time in between meals keeps both the glucose and the insulin high. This means that the body has no time to use up the energy that it has already stored in the liver or the fat tissue. Instead, the constant presence of insulin forces the cells of the body to keep storing more, and more, and more.

This is the point that health problems really start to take hold. Becoming obese is one thing. The extra weight may or may not affect you, but there comes a point when having extra fat starts the process of sickness.

We all know it. 'Fat' and 'sick' always seem to go together. It is such a common connection that we always assume it to be true.

Gaining weight, however, is just the start of the troubles. It is a sign of something else going on behind the scenes. You may not have been eating the '6-meals-a-day' routine, but you could be having multiple snacks, or just a general overconsumption of carbohydrate-filled foods. All these things keep insulin high.

When your body never gets to have that insulin down-time that it needs, the cells of your body begin to react differently – they start losing sensitivity to it. They start to ignore the presence of insulin, and one-by-one, the different types of cells become indifferent to its presence.

This has two devastating effects. One is that the cells begin to starve. Without insulin, there is no way for energy and nutrients to enter the cells. The second effect happens because the cells are not accepting food. As a result, the sugars and other particles continue to circulate with nowhere to go. This also means that there are a lot more particles to turn into fat. So, the liver turns it into fat, and the fat goes into storage somewhere.

This leads to a cascade of even more serious problems as we will see in a moment.

Excess Fat in Skinny People

Skinny people need to be just as mindful of their health, even if they find it impossible to add weight. Believe it or not, many thin people are so self-conscious of their 'skinny-ness' that they try all sorts of ways to add more weight on.

This is often a big mistake.

As a skinny guy, I also tried to add a few kilos of lean muscle mass by going to the gym. In fact, while I was at the gym, my weight didn't change at all for a long time, because there was extra fat sitting inside of me that slowly disappeared while my muscle mass increased.

Have you ever heard of TOFI? It stands for Thin on the Outside, Fat on the Inside. Many skinny people are actually fat on the inside, but just don't show it because fat does not build up anywhere else.

Inside-fat, also known as visceral fat, is the most dangerous type of fat. It is the type of fat that causes sickness, which means that skinny people are just as likely to develop acid reflux as those who are obese.

Many skinny people think that advice about weight does not apply to them. I am here to tell you differently. The health and weight information applies to you just as much as it applies to anyone with a weight that is greater than yours.

In fact, it may be more applicable. If you are skinny and you have already reached your fat capacity, then you need to take steps to deal with the problem. All the information that I am including about "obesity" applies just as much to you as anyone else!

The Answer to Obesity

You may be incredibly surprised to learn that the information I learned about fat and reflux came from a book about diabetes.

"Diabetes?" I hear you say. What about acid reflux? Why would someone like me be looking for information about acid reflux in a book about diabetes?

This is where things get interesting, because I first made the connection between diabetes and reflux through my own little discovery a few years earlier.

Most people are confused about the body. Why does the muscle at the top of the stomach (LES) become weak? Why does the stomach or the intestines slow down and not process food so quickly?

When people are looking for the greatest causes of reflux, they are normally looking at food 'triggers' and body weight, and nothing else about the disease makes any sense at all.

There is one enormous factor that nobody is taking about, and I think it is the single greatest cause of reflux disease on the planet. It causes most of the diseases that precede acid reflux, the diseases that accompany acid reflux disease, and it causes many of the complications that arise after reflux disease has taken hold.

It also contributes to weight gain. It is a beast that can keep a tight grip on your health and is involved with most of our modern diseases. If you can tame it, you can lower your inflammation and bring your weight back to its ideal level.

Let us look at what is probably the most important chapter in this book.

Testing for Inflammation

- See Appendix to chapter one for a list of possible tests

Further Reading

- *Life Without Diabetes* by Rod Taylor

CHAPTER 2

THE NUMBER ONE VILLAIN
OF REFLUX DISEASE

Have you ever wondered why some people get sick easily, or why some heal faster than others, age faster than others or why some people live in excellent health while other die early? One reason could be to do with genetics but that doesn't explain the sudden epidemics that we see in chronic diseases these days. Another reason could likely be insulin resistance.

Insulin resistance, or the loss of insulin sensitivity, sounds very tame, and you can imagine that it can lead to a few diseases down the track. But this is underestimating the condition.

It can cause or exacerbate small issues such as eczema, dermatitis, cold sores, or acne. Or it can cause muscle loss, or tinnitus, or launch you into heart failure, Alzheimer's, Parkinson's, or destroy your nervous system. Insulin resistance is the disease that leads to arm and leg amputations, blindness, and the heart-wrenching loss of memory that accompanies old age and cognitive decline.

It is the cause of most of the worst diseases that we consider to be chronic and incurable.

The sneaky part about insulin resistance is that you never realize you have it until it is too late. Most people go about their lives until one day, they suddenly discover that they have diabetes. They could have avoided the disease if they had detected the rise in insulin resistance 20 years earlier. With that enormous timeframe, for disease-in-the-making, imagine how many diseases could be prevented if we were to test for insulin resistance regularly!

As you read through this chapter, keep in mind that you already have insulin resistance too. Yes, you! You may not be aware of it yet, but the chances that you do not have it are close to zero. It may seem to be a bold statement to make, considering that I may not have even met you, but if you are reading this book because you have reflux, then you can be sure that some level of insulin resistance is involved.

Acid reflux sits along this insulin resistance timeline. On the bright side, acid reflux may be giving you a wake-up call, and forcing you to fix your health, because if you don't, then you may be on the way to further, more serious chronic diseases. Or maybe you have already been diagnosed with other diseases. Don't be surprised, because acid-reflux is never a solitary disease. There are always other diseases that accompany it.

And if you are reading this book, but you don't have reflux, then I can say with some confidence that you probably have insulin resistance, too. It may be a good idea to determine how the insulin resistance is manifesting itself in your body.

The reason that it applies to you is this. It is not a question about whether you will get it, but a question about whether you can ever escape it. Our modern world makes is almost impossible to stay completely healthy. Everybody is affected by it, and if you look up

WebMD it will tell you that, "…it is as widespread as pimples and the common cold." So, have you ever caught a cold? Is that a yes?

Take careful note of the information in this chapter because this is the primary cause of acid reflux. Not only is insulin resistance the greatest cause of reflux, but it has a hand in almost anything else that you may consider to be a cause of reflux. You will find insulin resistance is a strong theme that runs right through every chapter of this book.

What is Insulin Resistance?

The topic of insulin resistance has never really inspired a lot of research. The conditions that appear with insulin resistance were first described by Eskil Kylin in the 1920s, and over time it came to be known by several different names: Syndrome X, the insulin resistance syndrome, the deadly quartet, and obesity dyslipidemia syndrome.

These names all developed because different doctors in different places noticed that the same small cluster of diseases would all appear together, as if they were somehow linked. Let me give you 5 of them for starters:

- Diabetes
- Obesity
- Cholesterol imbalances
- High Blood Pressure
- Heart Disease

I'm not sure if you recognize this list of diseases, but they make up a cluster of diseases called "Metabolic Syndrome" (yet another name). The term Metabolic Syndrome was added to medical literature only in 1998, so it is something that was not officially recognized until recently.

So, what is the difference between Insulin Resistance and Metabolic Syndrome? The two are practically the same. Insulin Resistance is the cause of an entire spectrum of diseases and metabolic Syndrome is more specific to the small cluster of five diseases within that spectrum. Technically, insulin resistance is the cause of the metabolic syndrome diseases.

The name Metabolic Syndrome is very apt, because "Metabolic" refers to how our bodies process energy, and the term "syndrome" implies that there is something wrong with the way our bodies are processing the energy. It revolves around how we process sugars and fats for energy, as we saw in our discussion about insulin and other hormones in the previous chapter.

No one will ever have mentioned this to you, because metabolic syndrome does not have a defined range. It is an entire spectrum that ranges from absolutely perfect health all the way down to, umm, well... dead.

No coroner is going to announce 'insulin resistance' as a cause of death, but it is the insulin resistance that causes the terminal diseases. The point at which you experience reflux disease is far from the point of death. In fact, you may not have been diagnosed with any other serious diseases yet.

I always thought my skin problems - the eczema and rosacea - were just a small annoyance. I could control it to some extent, but I had no idea that those symptoms were connected to reflux and insulin resistance. I was never diagnosed with any of the five diseases listed above. It wasn't even close. Apart from the reflux, I thought that my health was great! I now know this was not the case. My reflux reflected my physical internal troubles.

Here is a small list of diseases that can be caused by insulin resistance, just to give you an idea of its impact:

- Metabolic Syndrome
  - Diabetes, etc, as listed previously

- Heart Disease
  - Hypertension
  - Vascular Diseases
  - Unhealthy blood lipids
  - Unbalance Cholesterol Profile
  - Atherosclerosis
  - Inflammation

- Neurological Disorders
  - Alzheimer's
  - Parkinson's
  - Vascular Dementia
  - Huntington's Disease
  - Migraines
  - Neuropathy (destruction of nerves)

- Reproductive Health
  - Gestational Diabetes
  - Pre-eclampsia (change in kidney function)
  - Over-and-underweight Babies
  - Low Breast Milk Supply
  - PCOS
  - Fertility in men and women
  - Low testosterone
  - Erectile dysfunction

Population studies have shown that half of us are insulin resistant, so it is not surprising that these diseases are all on the rise. And acid reflux is on the rise with them. The rise of acid reflux should not be surprising because of articles such as this one:

Increasing insulin resistance is associated with increased severity and prevalence of gastro-oesophageal reflux disease. (Aliment Pharmacol Ther. 2011 Oct;34(8):994-1004)

What this publication is saying, is that the worse your insulin resistance is, the worse your reflux will be.

Identifying Insulin Resistance

So, how can you know if you have insulin resistance? Here are a few examples of symptoms that could indicate insulin resistance:

- Weight gain, especially around the belly (internal organs).

- Dark patches of skin. This happens more in the areas where skin rubs together, like the armpits, groin etc.

- Skin tags (aka acrochoda). This comes from insulin over-stimulating the growth of the cells that provide structure to the skin.

- Psoriasis. Chronic inflammatory skin disease.

- Acne. People with acne have higher fasting levels of insulin.

- Tinnitus. People with this condition are highly likely to have insulin resistance or hyperinsulinemia.

- Muscle loss.

- Weak bones. People with insulin resistance may have normal bone mass, but the strength of the bones is reduced because the ongoing building and strengthening processes have slowed or stopped.

- Loss of cartilage in the joints.

- Loss of joint fluid (leading to rheumatoid arthritis).

- Gout. Insulin resistance causes the kidneys to keep uric acid rather than to excrete it.

These are just a few of the visible signs that you might see when insulin resistance is running at a level that is starting to affect you. Remember that I said it takes about 20 years for insulin resistance to develop into diagnosable diseases? Well, if you are experiencing symptoms like these, a number of those years have already past, and you are well on the way to developing other chronic diseases.

There are many reasons why insulin resistance can develop, or increase, and you may want to look at which factors are impacting your life already so that you can take steps to remove them.

Common Causes of Insulin Resistance

There are many factors that can increase your insulin resistance, and we don't have the space to discuss them in depth, so hold on to your seatbelt because we are going to take a very quick tour through the most common causes.

Don't get too caught up in the detail of it because we will address the nutritional ones and the lifestyle ones in books two and three. But this list will give you a heads-up on the types of things you should be looking out for.

When it comes to all the factors that can cause insulin resistance, inflammation is leader of the gang. It appears alongside other factors such as immune diseases, gut diseases, bacterial overgrowth, blood poisoning, visceral fat and a lot more. Unfortunately, inflammation is a very vague topic, because you can have a lot of inflammation that you don't even know about.

The best thing to do is to lower inflammation as much as possible, and we will be discussing the best step you can take for this, in the next chapter.

Oxidative stress is also a big contributor. It can be caused by obesity, consuming unhealthy fats, sugar, alcohol and certain medications, as well as tobacco products, pollution and exposure to pesticides or industrial chemicals.

Inside the body, these particles from these products interfere with chemical processes, and result in the manufacture of reactive oxygen species (ROS). These ROSs affect the internal working of the cells and impair the ability of cells to respond to insulin. The result is insulin resistance.

Air pollutants from our modern cities also incite inflammation. There are some studies that link air pollution with type 2 diabetes and insulin resistance. The most studied particle is PM2. It is so small that it can enter the lungs and make its way into the blood stream, and cause inflammation anywhere in the body. Even the larger particles such as PM10 can cause inflammation inside the lungs. The immune system detects them and sends out proteins that can cause a cascade of inflammatory processes.

Most cities give daily updates on the pollution particle readings. In many cases the information is available online.

Cigarette smoke is also one of the worst offenders, and as you probably know, it damages multiple organ systems and leads to various chronic diseases. Several studies have shown that cigarette smoke desensitizes the whole body to insulin, and this takes place after just the first cigarette.

Secondhand smoke, since it is unfiltered, is even more dangerous, triggering the release of lipid particles that are thought to be the main driver of smoking-related insulin resistance. And third-hand smoke – the chemicals that stick to clothing, hair and other surfaces – retains its ability to cause metabolic damage, especially for children that crawl or play with the clothing or hair of the adults.

Nicotine targets the fat cells to create insulin resistance. When fat cells become insulin resistant, the rest of the body tends to quickly follow suit. Switching to other nicotine products might seem like a good solution, but the evidence says otherwise. Nicotine gum tends to make insulin resistance worse than smoking the cigarette, and vaping is thought to be equally as bad as gum.

There are also many other chemicals that we absorb daily:

- MSG (monosodium glutamate) is a flavor enhancer that increases risk by 14% for every gram that is consumed.

- Petrochemicals that are found in clothing, lotions, foods and drink (including BPA) tend to cause insulin resistance.

- Pesticides are highly correlated with insulin resistance. Pesticides tend to accumulate in fat stores, especially visceral fat which can store ten times more than subcutaneous fat.

- Artificial sweeteners are not the great sugar alternative, as we are told in the media. Sugars such as glucose and fructose can cause insulin resistance and oxidative stress, but artificial sweeteners taken daily can lead to a huge increase in the risk for developing metabolic syndrome (36%) and diabetes (67%).

And the worst toxins of all are Lipopolysaccharides (LPS). These molecules are everywhere – in the air, in our food and our drinks. But the most relevant source of these toxins is from specific types of bacteria, known as gram-negative bacteria. These bacteria have a protective cell membrane made of LPS. These types of bacteria can be good or bad, but when the bacteria die, the LPS molecules continue to float about. If they are killed off in large amounts in the intestines, they can cause diarrhea and inflammation. This leads to gut permeability, and the ability for the molecules to enter the bloodstream.

Inside the body they can cause many severe health effects, including the activation of inflammation throughout the body. The immune system is also activated which can heighten the inflammatory effects. They are detectable in the blood, and they have been found in higher amounts in people who are insulin resistant and those that are overweight.

The body does have one remarkably effective defense against LPS, and that is LDL cholesterol, traditionally labelled as the 'bad' cholesterol. LDL carries a special protein called "LPS-binding-protein". The cholesterol physically binds to the LPS. From there it travels to the liver, where it is passed to the intestines and out of the body. LDL cholesterol plays a significant role in fighting infections, which may be why those with low LDL cholesterol levels are more likely to experience severe infections.

By way of diet, the obvious contributor to insulin resistance is sugar, sweet foods and carbohydrates. Those ones are well known, but the one you may not have heard about is salt. The problem arises in those that are eating too little salt, not too much. When salt levels are too low in the body, the kidneys respond by releasing a hormone that does two things – it helps to conserve salt in the blood, and it blocks the action of insulin, adding to insulin resistance. Living a lifestyle that is salt-free is extremely unhealthy for many reasons, and studies have already linked low salt consumption to diseases such as heart disease.

And one final remark about fasting. This practice is becoming increasingly popular these days, which is great. The problem arises when fasting is not carried out properly. There is a definite line between fasting and starvation. Fasting uses body-fat for fuel whereas starvation is the tendency for the body to break down muscle tissue to be able to feed itself. The point at which that line is crossed depends very much from person to person, but during starvation, insulin resistance sets in.

Thoughts on Lowering Insulin Resistance

In the following chapter we will discuss the primary, single most effective way to deal with insulin resistance, that is, low-carb diets. Although this style of eating can be incredibly effective, there is certainly more than one way to increase your chances of raising your sensitivity to insulin. Here are a few ideas.

Exercise. Sedentary living is the highway to hell if we are talking about chronic disease. Everyone knows that a lack of activity is unhealthy. In terms of insulin resistance, just one week without any activity can increase insulin resistance seven-fold. And insulin sensitivity doesn't just return if you begin being active again. Resistance to insulin tends to last for a long period of time after you begin exercising again.

Sleep. Just one week with not enough sleep can increase insulin resistance by up to 30%, compared to a week of normal sleep. The amount of sleep each person needs varies, so this is something that each person needs to work out for themselves. But on the other hand, napping too much can also cause increased insulin resistance. People who nap more than one hour a day are more likely to develop insulin resistance than those that only nap for about 30 minutes.

Fasting. There are lots of different ways to fast, but when it is done properly, and regularly, fasting can boost your insulin sensitivity significantly. When the body is well adjusted with the correct diets, fasting can become easy. It is good to fast occasionally for a few days at a time, but most people engage in much more regular fasting for shorter periods, often daily, for 12 to 20 hours.

Vitamins and Minerals. Nutritional aspects can have a great impact on our health. The foods that make up a standard Western diet cause so much wastage of vitamins and minerals, that it is hardly surprising that so many people struggle so much with their health. Magnesium is needed by insulin receptors to work properly, so when this mineral is in deficit, insulin resistance is inevitable. The diets in the next chapter will certainly help with this regard, but we will talk more about vitamins and minerals in more depth in the sections dedicated to nutrition.

Reduce Stress. Stress changes the body's chemistry to keep it prepared for sudden maneuvers, such as the type that you might get in a chase or when fleeing from predators. In these times, the blood sugar in the body rises, and hormones are released to give your energy levels a boost. The hormones that are released are generally responsible for the decrease in insulin sensitivity. Under normal circumstances, this stress would normally be short-lived, but in our modern society, stress is an everyday occurrence, leading to increased insulin resistance and massive declines in health.

How I Discovered Insulin-Resistance/Acid-Reflux Connection

When I discovered that acid reflux was related to insulin resistance, I was very shocked, to say the least, and I only discovered the link because I was researching low carb information. I went from discovering low-carb diets, and then on to ketogenic diets which are very well-researched. This was just before ketogenic diets went on to become hugely popular, but there was still a lot of scientific information available, at the time.

I was astounded at the number of diseases that ketogenic diets were supposed to cure (we will visit the ketogenic diet in the next chapter). There was toenail fungus, acid-reflux disease, digestive issues, all the way up to brain diseases. And, to boot, it would fix all your weight-loss issues too!

The information I discovered was revealing to me, because I began to recognize the relationship between all the diseases that ran through my family.

From Alzheimer's in my great-grandmother, dementia and glaucoma in my grandfather, to various other ailments in their children. That was on my mother's side, and then on my father's side, all the different forms of metabolic syndrome were rampant and highly visible. Diabetes and Heart disease were the big ones.

During my researching, I came across a couple of articles about the link between acid reflux and insulin resistance (metabolic syndrome and diabetes).

The Headlines were:

Insulin Resistance in Gastroesophageal Reflux Disease (Acta Med Indones. 2018 Oct;50(4):336-342)

High prevalence of gastroesophageal reflux symptoms in type 2 diabetics… (Nutr Metab (Lond). 2012 Jan 25;9(1):4)

Gastroesophageal reflux and metabolic syndrome (Rev Med Chir Soc Med Nat Iasi. Jul-Sep 2013;117(3):605-9)

At the time, I was flabbergasted! Why was this information hidden and unknown? Why had I never heard about it? It was sitting there in plain sight, but no one seemed to know about it. And the solution to acid reflux was also there, because in that last journal article, I read through the summary. And the conclusion said exactly this: "We consider that treatment of reflux disease in these particular cases must also involve measures to correct metabolic disorders."

If you want to overcome reflux disease, you must correct any metabolic disorders. And this has been our discussion throughout this chapter.

This was my first step into understanding many of the true causes of acid reflux. This is why this discussion about insulin resistance and metabolic syndrome is so important. Moving on from here we must talk about metabolic diets. These can fix many metabolic disorders. Metabolic diets, in combination with other strategies, can give you a lifestyle that is incredibly effective at sensitizing your cells to insulin.

Note: Any mention of diabetes in this chapter (and throughout this book, unless specified) refers to Diabetes Type II. In contrast, diabetes type I is an autoimmune disease and not a lifestyle disease and needs to be treated differently.

What You Can Do

Supplements that help reduce insulin resistance

- Magnesium

- Chromium Picolinate has been shown to reduce insulin resistance and reduce carb cravings.

- Sunlight and vitamin D

- Good quality vitamin B complex

Lifestyle

- Spend a short amount of time each day walking.

Testing for Insulin Resistance

- HOMA-IR Test for insulin resistance

- Cholesterol and blood panel test to find any irregularities

Further Reading

- *Why We Get Sick* by Benjamin Bikman

CHAPTER 3

THE TRUE REFLUX-REDUCING DIET

I used to eat extremely healthy meals. I used to receive comments regularly about how healthy my food looked – lots of vegetables and fruit, healthy whole grains. I would eat brown rice instead of white rice, and brown bread instead of white bread. But it was all wrong for reflux. I talk about the reasons why in book two, but discovering the correct diet is one of the most important steps in overcoming acid reflux.

Whenever I am asked what the single most effective step is for combatting reflux is, my answer is always this: A Low Carb Metabolic Diet! This is, hands-down, the single most powerful and effective step you can take to curing reflux disease. This is the step you should take before removing acid-reflux medications, and it is the step that you absolutely must be doing before any other step can become effective.

It is important to note that this diet is not a weight loss diet. It is a weight-balancing diet that should be followed by both thin and overweight people alike. If you are too thin, it can bring you to your ideal weight and improve your health, and if you are overweight, it can bring you to your ideal weight and improve your health.

It does this, not because of calorie restriction (low calorie diets are extremely unhealthy), but because it balances the hormones that run the metabolism in your system. It is our hormones, and not calories, that determine our weight. Our modern diets and lifestyles keep our hormones out of whack, but when hormones are balanced, then everything you are looking for begins to fall into place.

Most people that have acid reflux are willing to follow all sort of very strange and extreme diets. I did, out of sheer desperation. But in most cases, these diets are the wrong ones! Unfortunately, they are designed to 'manage' reflux, and not to cure it. For many years I went through the same procedures. It is tiring because you need to constantly re-evaluate the ingredients that you are eating, but in the end the underlying problems remain, despite all the effort.

It is because of low carb eating (and the steps in later chapters) that I can now eat oranges, chocolate, and have regular coffees, and occasional drinks. I even eat a bag of chocolate-coated coffee beans on occasion without complaint. But without this diet, this could never have happened.

Is this Diet for Everyone?

Is this diet one-size-fits-all? Absolutely not! For a start, it is not just one diet. You have loads of flexibility. And secondly, this style of eating is a foundational principle. You must pass through this gate before your reflux woes can be properly dealt with.

If you have ever heard anyone say that a low carb diet didn't work for them, you can be sure that they have not understood the concept. There is not just one way to follow low carb. In fact, in this chapter I am going to introduce you to three different ways to follow low carb eating.

And this is not going to be the end of your dieting journey. What I am introducing to you here is something that you are going to build upon, because in book two of this series, we will be discussing specific factors in your diet that affect how your diet works for you. At that stage you will learn some information that can make an enormous difference to your success. And you will be able to test these things for yourself.

A low carb lifestyle will help you to discover what improves your metabolism and what makes it worse.

At the end of this chapter, and when you get to know some basic principles of low carb diets, you will be able to identify some of the faults in other anti-reflux diets and figure out why many people don't respond to them so well.

How I Encountered Low-Carb Diets

A lot of people have hesitations about following low-carb diets. Thinking about all the favorite foods that they will have to give up on this diet often sounds like a death-sentence. My own experience of starting low carb was just the opposite. I thought I would only be on low carb levels for a short time, so the commitment level seemed a lot smaller. Let me share my story with you.

A number of years ago, in my ongoing search for answers to my health issues, I visited a naturopathic physician. At the time, my gut health was a priority, and this woman was supposed to be an expert in gut health.

As part of the process, we wanted to make sure that gut bugs were not the cause of any of the issues, so she started me on a small program that would help my body to clear them. As part of the program, she instructed me to change to a low-carb diet for the next four weeks. This was to ensure that the natural medications would work, and that I was not feeding the gut bugs too much.

At the time, I was close to devastated about having to take this on. I was trying to add some bulk at the gym, and as it was, I was struggling. It was difficult enough to get through the exercises at each gym-day, and my progress week-to-week seemed incredibly slow. I was always told that carbohydrates gave you energy to burn, so I was hesitant to lower my carb intake. Would it make my gym progress even worse? Would I go backwards after all the weeks I had spent there?

I decided to go ahead with the program, and I cut the carbs from my food. I was supposed to limit my carbohydrate intake to 130g per day, but when I calculated how much I was eating, it was easily 600g or 700g per day! Being the lazy person that I am, there was no way that I was going to sit there all day long calculating carbohydrate levels in food. I couldn't be bothered. Instead, I simply cut out all the foods that obviously contained carbs and continued to eat all the foods that contained next to no carbohydrates at all. I didn't calculate my food levels, but I was definitely eating well under 130g each day.

I expected to start feeling run-down generally, and exhausted at the gym. But the effect was exactly the opposite, and an enormous surprise. At the gym, I was powering through all the exercises. The pain couldn't hold me back. I loved it! And every single week, without fail, I had to increase the weights. I had never made so much progress so quickly.

Outside the gym, I felt amazing, and I had loads of energy to burn. As the weeks rolled by, I considered the difference that low carb had made for me. After experiencing so much improvement, I didn't want to go back to feeing the way I was. I knew that carbohydrates were causing me to lose my life, and as the fourth week was coming to an end, I decided that I was never going to eat carbs again.

I had no idea whether this sort of eating was supposed to be healthy, especially long-term, but I was ready to do some research. Little did I know that this would be the beginning of my new health journey that led me to where I am today.

Benefits of a Metabolic Diet

The benefits you will experience on this diet are extensive. I couldn't possibly provide a comprehensive list, but I'll try to explain the main benefits throughout the next few chapters. However, here are a few benefits to give you some idea to begin with:

- Eliminates bloating
- Combats intestinal infections
- Combats skin infections
- Combats or cures depression
- Protects nerves, veins and digestive system functions
- Reverses insulin resistance and inflammation
- Allows easier removal of PPI drugs
- Weight loss for overweight people
- Weight redistribution for skinny people
- Protection from Barrett's Esophagus and gastroparesis

One factor that I have seen reported is the development of Barrett's Esophagus, even in those taking PPI medications. That was on a conventional acid-reflux diet, so I am happy to report that this type of diet can not only improve health but also protect from the biggest threats to the health of reflux sufferers.

Let's take a look at the factors that make this diet so effective for reflux:

- Fixes the specific weight issues that cause reflux
- Increases insulin sensitivity
- Balances hormones (to balance weight)
- Reduces pathogens in the gut that increase reflux symptoms
- Reduces inflammation and other related causes of reflux
- Improves your body's immune system

Understanding the Low Carb Approach

Low-carb diets are based on cutting down on one macronutrient: Carbohydrates. There are three main components to food: protein, fat, and carbohydrate. Protein is found mainly in meats and animal products, but there is also a small amount of protein in some plant foods as well. Fats are found in both animal and plant foods, and carbohydrates, apart from milk and honey, are normally only found in plant foods.

I have three low-carb diet approaches that I want to share with you. There are also a few things that you need to know before jumping into a low-carb diet, so let us look at the three approaches first, and then we will discuss what you need to know before you begin.

Cautionary Note

Many people on modern diets end up on medications such as metformin. These drugs are simply forcing our bodies to do something that should be happening naturally, such as balancing blood-sugar levels. If you are on any medications at all, you must see a doctor before beginning a low-carb diet, because the combined effect of the diet and the medication could cause serious harm.

Low Carb Diet 1 – General Low Carb

A little confusing... but the name low-carb can be applied to any diet where carbohydrates are cut down, including ketogenic diets (or very-low carb diets), and even zero-carb.

As a diet style of its own, a low-carb diet consists of this one single principle:

"Eat less than 130g of carbohydrates per day."

It is as simple as that. But if this type of diet style is new to you, it may take some time to figure out how much 130g is going to be. If you are lazy like me, you probably won't want to measure food quantities. Instead, look up some charts to gauge how many carbs are in your usual foods, and then just cut out all the foods that are obviously high-carb foods:

- Bread
- Pasta
- Pastries
- Rice
- Anything made with grains
- Sweet foods
- Potatoes and sweet potatoes
- Most fruits
- Anything that grows under the ground

A low-carb diet gives you a lot of room to move if you want to indulge in something sweet, like some fruits, but remember that if you do this, you will need to start counting how many carbs you are eating each day. It is easy to go over the limit.

When taking up a low carb diet follow these pieces of advice also:

- Check the carb content of all foods. You don't want to go over your limit.

- Avoid vegetable oil like the plague.

- Make sure you eat salt. Don't cut this out. Make your food taste good.

- Eat whole foods, not commercially prepared products of any sort.

- Beware of prepared sauces. Avoid them if you can. They are normally high in sugar.

- Don't be afraid to eat healthy fats. Without carbs, fats can be eaten liberally. These can include the fats naturally found in foods, such as fatty steaks, or avocados and from some cold-pressed plants such as coconut oil and olive oil.

And because we are dealing with reflux, it would be better to avoid these foods for now:

- Dairy products
- Drinking coffee or too much coffee
- Raw vegetables and excess fibrous food (for gut health)
- Excessive protein consumption

Regarding fats, unfortunately, many people over many years train themselves to develop a distaste to natural fats in our foods. In addition to this, most people are led to believe that fats cause reflux. On the other hand, don't go overboard with your fat consumption at this stage. We will visit this topic more thoroughly in book two.

It is often easiest to start off by eating the same types of foods that you are used to, minus the carb-filled parts. Here are some examples:

- Salad sandwiches: Remove the bread so that the meal becomes a salad. Or wrap the ingredients inside a lettuce leaf.

- Indian curries: Remove the carbohydrate portion which is rice. The meal will become just the curry sauce with the chunky ingredients, such as meat. If you decide to include rice, make sure the carbohydrate quantity does not bring you over your daily carb allowance. Also, do not use a commercial sauce – it will be full of sugars and other harmful ingredients.

- Stir Fries are a good option. They generally use a broad range of vegetables that are all low carb. Simply remove the carbohydrate-rich side portions of the meal such as rice.

Salt is important. If there is a particular reason you do not want to eat more salt, read about salt in the section on Nutrition, and see a doctor before you start.

In general, going low carb really is extremely easy. Although 130g of carbs sounds like a tough limit, once you get used to the range of foods you can eat and the ways to prepare them, you won't feel deprived at all.

Low Carb Diet 2 - Ketogenic Diet (Very Low Carb)

A very low carb diet is a ketogenic diet.

This type of diet is very specific in only one sense: Your body must begin producing ketones.

The name of the diet comes from the special compounds created by the liver, called ketones. The liver converts fats into compounds called 'ketones', which are then used by the body's cells for energy. Since ketones are only produced under these special dietary conditions, any diet that allows production of ketones can be known as a ketogenic diet, whether that is a very low carb diet, a zero carb diet, a meat-only diet or even a ketogenic version of a paleo diet.

Ketogenic diets have become very popular in the last few years, mainly due to their strength in aiding weight loss. The diet calls for the consumption of very high levels of fat and very low levels of carbohydrate. This particular food combination triggers the body's natural fat-burning mechanism, and relies on the body's ability to use fats for energy instead of sugars.

In order to bring your body into this state of 'ketosis', your carbohydrate consumption must be low enough to allow this process to begin. The level of carbohydrates you can eat to achieve this will depend on the health of your body, but a good guideline is to eat less than 20g of carbohydrates per day.

This cuts down your food choices a lot! So, you will need to start planning. To get going on a ketogenic diet, you will need some tools, and you will need to keep your food in specific proportions to make the diet work effectively.

Tools you will need

The first thing you need to do is to buy a meter for measuring ketones in your system. And you will need a computer/phone app, or some sort of food-list that can tell you the macronutrient breakdown of the foods that you are eating.

Ketostix can give you an indication of when you are beginning to produce ketones. They are very inexpensive strips that measure ketones in your urine, but they are just a rough guide. They will get you started on this diet but will probably only last for a month before they stop working. Once your body gets used to using ketones for energy, it stops excreting them in the urine, so the Ketostix will register a false negative result.

The best indicator of your ketone levels is the blood-sugar/ketone meter that diabetics use. They are a little more expensive, but it will be able to give you an exactly accurate indication of how you are going. It also tells you how much sugar is in your blood, which can also be helpful.

If these tools are showing that you are not producing ketones, you may need to re-evaluate your food choices.

There are many, many apps out there that count macronutrients: carbohydrates, proteins and fats. You can google these or search for an app that will give you the information that you need. You can also consult the list that is on the website for readers of this book. Just go to **www.acidrefluxformula.com/book-1-additional-material**

Macronutrient Proportions (daily amounts)

In order to achieve ketosis, you will need to limit your macronutrient portions to specific amounts.

- Carbohydrates portion (daily): 20g

- Protein portion: between 50g and 150g depending on your ideal weight (see below)

- Fat portion: Unlimited amounts. This makes up the rest of the calories for the day

On a ketogenic diet, you need to know your protein requirements. You can do this by calculating your ideal weight for your height (might not be your current weight) and multiplying that by 0.36 if the weight is in pounds or multiplying by 0.8 if the weight is in kilograms. The result will give the number of grams of protein you can eat. For example, a woman that weighs 140 pounds will be able to eat 50g of protein. This is the minimum. The maximum is roughly double that amount but remember that too much protein can keep you out of a ketogenic state. Don't overdo it on protein. It may take some experimentation to determine your ideal level.

This diet is a high-fat diet, so in your caloric needs for the day, after your low carbohydrate calories and your moderate protein calories, the rest of your daily calorie needs are made up with fats. It is a very satisfying way to eat.

This can be a scary concept for many people with reflux, but the truth is that when the correct fats are taken in the correct way, they can improve your reflux condition, not make it worse. Fat intake needs to be in the context of a ketogenic diet (not just any diet), and the fats need to be healthy ones (not vegetable oils!). You can learn much more about how the body uses fats in book two.

Food Choices

Here is what you must avoid:

- All grains and grain products
- All sweet foods
- All root vegetables
- All fruits (except a few low-carb versions)
- Dairy (except butter and ghee)

Here is what you can eat:

- Low-carb vegetables
- Meats, up to your protein limit
- Eggs (check protein limit)
- Healthy fats, eg. Lard, Tallow, Coconut oil, Olive Oil

There is a difficulty with dairy that I will discuss in book two, but for now, just remember that it would be best to avoid dairy for the best results.

For most people, a ketogenic diet comes as a breath of fresh air - something that makes dieting easy, gives you lots of energy, and makes you feel great!

For other people, a ketogenic diet, with all its benefits, is just another exercise in great self-discipline, causing constant cravings for more food, and more carbohydrates.

I was in the latter group. For me, the standard ketogenic diet really fixed the bulk of my reflux problems. But it left me always craving more food. And that was not the only difficulty I had with it. The food choices did not make life with my gut easy, and I don't believe that the foods people eat on a ketogenic diet is incredibly healthy, even if they are natural, because most choices are high in histamines, oxalates and salicylates, among other things, and this was my biggest issue with the standard ketogenic diet.

I'll be talking a lot about food choices in the nutrition section in book two, and which ones can make a big difference to your health.

And to be clear, there is a lot to be gained from a ketogenic diet. There is a lot of science behind ketogenic diets, and it is freely available. I will leave it to you to do the research that you want to do. It is known to clear up reflux, food intolerances and a whole swathe of health issues, both minor and major.

Low Carb Diet 3 – Zero Carb Diet

A zero-carb diet is a subset of what is commonly known as a carnivore diet. It is completely free of any plant foods and consists mainly of meat as well as other zero-carb animal products, such as eggs.

Foods such as milk and honey contain carbohydrates, so although some carnivore diets include these foods, a zero-carb diet does not.

The difference with zero carb is not just the lack of plants, which almost all contain carbohydrates of some sort. You also remove all the toxins and fiber that tend to wreak havoc with the intestines of so many people. When your intestinal lining needs extra care, removing these foods can make all the difference.

Many people have doubts about following such a diet, and I was no exception. After all, isn't it dangerous to stop eating plants? In fact, red meat was one of the foods that I was apparently intolerant to. I would develop skin problems if I ate red meat, which was confirmed in an elimination diet. And an allergy test also showed that I was probably intolerant to it.

Like most people, I was definitely influenced by the common rumors about nutrition. My biggest concerns about the diet were these:

- Are plants needed to avoid constipation?
- Isn't eating red meat bad for you?
- Where do you get your vitamins and minerals if you only eat meat?
- Isn't a meat-only diet boring?

Fortunately, group discussions provided the answers to these problems. It turns out that plants are the greatest cause of constipation, and this has been demonstrated in some small studies. Red meat can be bad for you if you eat it as burgers and other processed forms, whereas, in its natural form, as steaks, it is perfectly healthy. In fact, red meat (muscle meat) is the most nutrient dense food on the planet, after organ meats (such as liver), and it is much more easily absorbed than most plant foods.

And is it boring to eat just meat? Well, think of it as indulging in your favorite food, day-in and day-out. You become accustomed to the variety of flavors in the different meats, and when I get hungry, all I can think about is tucking into my favorite meat dish.

At the time when I had trouble with a standard ketogenic diet, I considered my options carefully. I knew I had to stay low carb. I didn't want to go back to the way I felt on a standard western high-carb diet. I had started on a low-carb diet, and that was an amazing experience. Progressing to a ketogenic diet had given me even more benefits, but it caused me a lot of anguish with bowel problems (constipation!).

Switching to a carnivore diet was the best thing I ever did! Starting a low-carb diet for the first time was an amazing experience, but starting carnivore was even better! The energy and mental clarity it gave me was what I was looking for in the other two diets.

Starting on a carnivore diet does not come without its problems, though. This is something that I discovered. Although eating meat-only sounds simple, if you have been suffering from reflux and digestive complaints of any sort, I have a few tips that can help make life easier. You will find these pointers in the appendix section.

Final Thoughts

If you are not familiar with low-carb diets, the rules can seem a bit overwhelming. But take heart. These types of diets are extremely popular, so there is no lack of information on the topic, and you will have no trouble finding people to talk to about the subject.

A low carb diet is essential to beating reflux. The next steps rely heavily on the effect that a low carb diet will have on your body, so make sure you have been on this type of diet for about two weeks before moving on to the next step. It takes some time to adapt to a low carb diet properly.

When you have achieved this, the process of stepping down from PPI medications and fixing your gut in the up-coming chapter should be a breeze.

Further Diet Instructions

- See the appendix to chapter three for more information on following very-low-carb and zero-carb diets.

Further Reading

- Any book about how to follow a ketogenic diet. There are many!

- *Fat of the Land*, by Vilhjalmur Stefansson

- *The Carnivore Diet*, by Shawn Baker

- Zerocarbzen.com

CAUTION!

- See low carb doctor, especially if you are on medications.

- Low carb diets can replace sugar-lowering medications but do not take these medications while on a low carb diet.

CHAPTER 4

ELIMINATING REFLUX MEDICATION

Now that you have some low carb diets underway, it is time to think about making some changes. Medication can often feel like a ball and chain on your life, so dropping the reflux medications can provide some freedom in multiples ways. If you want to kick reflux, then you must stop taking anti-acid drugs. Without taking this step, it will be impossible for you to overcome acid reflux disease.

The drugs that I want to focus on are Proton Pump Inhibitors (PPI), because these are the most prescribed and are the most potent. There are several other drugs that affect stomach acid levels, and these are safer for your health but remember that it is never a good idea to combat reflux by lowering stomach acid levels.

Did you know that PPIs tend to make reflux worse? Instead of helping and solving the problem of reflux, PPI medications increase the severity of reflux over time.

There are three especially important points that we need to know about PPI drugs so that we can understand why this is the case.

Firstly, they do not treat the problem. PPIs are not designed to fix reflux. They are only designed to stop the stomach from producing acid. The reflux from the stomach continues to happen, but you may not notice because there is no longer any acid to trigger the pain. There are certainly legitimate and practical uses for PPI medications, but curing acid reflux is not one of them.

Secondly, they can cause many diseases if you are taking them for more than a few weeks. The long-term effects are becoming very well-known and widely publicized. The side effects include everything from increased susceptibility to flus and pneumonia, to intestinal infections, nutritional deficiencies, osteoporosis, cardiovascular disease, stroke, dementia and autoimmune disease. And if you add in complications that can arise from those diseases, then the list gets much longer.

Thirdly, they make the causes of reflux worse. PPIs are used to mask the main symptoms of reflux disease, not to fix it. And in addition to this, the lack of acid creates and exacerbates the long-term diseases such as gut and stomach infections that can make reflux even worse over time.

In short, the longer you are on PPI medications, the more damage you may be doing to your body, and the worse your underlying reflux disease can become. It is important to know that some types of damage such as kidney failure or stroke are not reversible, and in addition, it is more difficult to give up PPIs the longer you have been taking them.

The best thing to do, in my opinion, is to remove the PPI drugs, and to fix the real causes of reflux instead.

It was not too many years ago that PPI medications were thought to be completely safe. These days, the long list of side effects are listed on the leaflet that comes with the medication and more people are starting to ask questions about the safety of the drugs.

It is good to note also that the U.S. Food and Drug Administration issued warnings in 2011 advising that over-the-counter PPIs should be used for no longer than two weeks at a time for up to three treatments per year. This warning is still current on their website at the time of writing: **https://www.fda.gov/drugs/postmarket-drug-safety-information-patients-and-providers/fda-drug-safety-communication-possible-increased-risk-fractures-hip-wrist-and-spine-use-proton-pump**

Let's quickly highlight some of the most common health complaints associated with PPI usage, and then have a look at how to step down off of PPI drugs.

PPIs Are Toxic to Your Gut Health

The most common reflux advice these days aims to ensure that food in your stomach is digested as soon as possible, so that your stomach can empty into the intestines. An empty stomach is less likely to cause reflux. It also aims to limit bad gut bacteria that cause bloating and intestinal problems.

PPI drugs, on the other hand, do just the opposite.

One of the major effects that PPI drugs have on the gastrointestinal system is to slow it down. Firstly, it slows down gastric emptying, so that food remains in the stomach longer. Secondly, it slows down the intestinal system, and thirdly, it reduces the thickness of mucus on the stomach walls.

All three of these effects are known to cause acid reflux. So as soon as you begin to take PPI drugs, the problems can begin to compound. Remember, if the drugs are blocking acid production, then you may not feel the pain of the extra reflux episodes.

The reduction in speed of the system, and the thinning of mucus have a number of effects.

Firstly, it makes the intestines even more comfortable for pathogens. The lack of movement gives more time for these microbes to grow and take up residence anywhere in the gut. It also creates abnormal bacterial counts in the large intestine and can cause SIBO (bacterial overgrowth) in the small intestines.

The next most common symptom, diarrhea, follows on from bacterial overgrowth. A slow-down in gut movement will normally cause constipation, but the experience of most people is just the opposite. The build-up of pathogens produces toxic biproducts which result in an ongoing case of diarrhea.

If you are unlucky enough to develop a case of dysbiosis like this, it could take months or years to overcome this completely. This was my experience which I will share in the next chapter on fixing the gut.

Also be aware that if you already suffer from gastric or intestinal disease such as IBS, IBD or Crohn's disease, then long-term PPI medications could make your condition much worse. This is just the beginning of the health decline that has been observed and studied with PPI use.

PPIs accelerate H.Pylori damage

H.Pylori is a bacteria that inhabits the human stomach, and has been a part of our existence for thousands of years. It confers benefits for our health in many ways, but if it is left unchecked, it can cause damage to the lining of the stomach.

The body has its ways of keeping H.Pylori in line. One of those is the acidity of the stomach. Yes, H.Pylori can live in acidic environments, but it is still not the easiest environment for it to thrive and proliferate. When the acid level drops with PPIs, H.Pylori populations can grow out of control.

Studies have shown that taking PPI mediations while H.Pylori is present can increase the risk of developing atrophic gastritis. Atrophic gastritis can lead to stomach cancer, so taking PPI medications when H.Pylori is present increases that risk substantially. However, it is unknown whether PPI drugs can cause atrophic gastritis over long periods of time on its own, without the help of other factors.

Other PPI-related cancer

Another debated cause of stomach cancer is through the proliferation of other microbes (other than H.Pylori) in the stomach. PPI medications lower or eliminate acid in the stomach, allowing other microbes to move in. These bacteria can produce nitrites from natural compounds in foods. Nitrites are carcinogenic compounds and are found in higher concentrations in people who have little to no stomach acid.

Rises in stomach cancer have been documented with the use of PPI drugs. However, the studies failed to eliminate other cancer-causing factors. This is what makes the PPI-Cancer connection debatable. But would you take the chance if you're given the choice?

PPIs drain your electrolytes

One of the most important elements for day-to-day function of your body are electrolytes. Electrolytes are needed in the body for optimal health and for thousands of different chemical reactions that take place constantly. In fact, electrolytes can directly affect various functions of your gut, including the nerves and the muscles. These electrolytes include magnesium, calcium and potassium.

Research is identifying magnesium deficiency as an emerging global health crisis. Magnesium deficiency is a feature in many illnesses, but in those treated for reflux disease, PPI drugs make the situation much worse. Low magnesium levels lead to low levels of calcium and potassium, so in one foul swoop, PPI medications can rob you of the electrolytes that are essential to cell function and to hundreds of reactions that need to take place in your body to support the functions of your gut. Studies have found that magnesium levels are not just low in patients on PPI medication, but they are *severely* low in 97% of these patients.

Magnesium is an electrolyte that is linked to overcoming reflux disease, not only through the gut but also through other bodily processes that magnesium maintains for good health. This means that PPI drugs are likely to put the brakes on your recovery from acid reflux disease. Magnesium helps your muscles and nervous system to relax, so that digestion improves. On the other hand, a magnesium deficiency causes severe digestive trouble because it makes the pyloric sphincter remain tight (hypertension), leading to gastroparesis, where the stomach cannot move its contents into the intestines.

Low levels of magnesium almost always lead to low levels of calcium. This is because a lack of magnesium down regulates the parathyroid gland which is involved in maintaining proper calcium levels in the system.

Calcium is needed by your nervous system for impulse transmission and for proper muscle function. It is also essential for organs and cells. A lack of it results in muscle cramps and spasms, muscle weakness and tingling in the extremities. It is also involved in the production of hormones, and it is important in maintaining the integrity of your gut lining. All these factors are involved in how your gut moves and how food is processed, so low calcium could cause a lot of gastrointestinal distress.

Many antacids are involved in reducing calcium levels because they contain aluminum hydroxide. Not only does aluminum cause constipation, but aluminum can also cause calcium loss, making the intestinal situation even worse.

Low Magnesium levels also lead to low potassium levels. Low potassium can also lead to muscle cramps and weakness. It can cause nausea and vomiting and can cause partial paralysis of the intestines. It is also important in the stomach where it helps with the production and secretion of acid, to improve the digestion of the foods we eat.

And lastly, proper magnesium levels can improve insulin sensitivity. It has been shown to help with diabetes and to reduce that incidence of atherosclerosis which leads to heart disease. This is good news for anyone that is trying to reverse insulin resistance.

PPIs reduce your body's vitamins and minerals

Other vitamins and minerals can also have a significant impact on your reflux symptoms.

B12 is a vitamin that is important for the neurological system including the brain and nerves. A lack of B12 can cause depression, memory loss and behavioral changes, weakness and fatigue, and nerve problems. Nerve problems might be felt through tingling or numbness, but it can also affect the entire gastrointestinal system leading to reflux, as well as abdominal bloating, constipation, diarrhea and a loss of appetite.

Zinc is also important for fighting reflux symptoms. Even a mild deficiency in zinc can cause many diseases that lead to reflux: chronic inflammatory diseases such as cirrhosis, inflammatory bowel disease and chronic pancreatitis. It leaves the body open to infections and animal studies have suggested that it can lead to cancer of the esophagus. Raising zinc levels reverses the danger of developing esophageal tumors.

Iron can also be affected over long periods of time – iron-deficiency anemia can result in fatigue, cognitive impairment, neurodegeneration, thyroid issues and lowered ability to fight infections. These last two symptoms can affect the gut directly. Malfunction of the thyroid gland can cause low stomach acid output and can make the whole gastrointestinal system to become sluggish. And without being able to fight infections, the intestines are likely to succumb to attack from all sorts of microbes, leading to inflammation and possible damage to the gut lining.

It is also good to mention that folate levels can be affected. This may be more of a danger for those that are experiencing growth such as infants, adolescents and pregnant women. Folate is involved in the production of blood cells in the bone marrow, and it is also important for the construction of DNA and RNA. If stomach acid is not stronger than a pH of 4.0, the body may not be able to absorb enough of this vitamin.

Insulin Resistance

When I first found out about insulin resistance, I noticed that many of the diseases caused by PPI drugs overlapped with those caused by insulin resistance, but there was never any study on the subject. But then, in 2020, an observational study suggested that it can increase a patient's risk of developing type 2 diabetes by 24% if they were taking PPI two or more times per week. [*Regular use of proton pump inhibitors and risk of type 2 diabetes* (Gut. 2021 Jun;70(6):1070-1077)]

Previously, diabetes and insulin resistance were not thought to be a risk factor in PPI use, but this was because no one had investigated the link with the drugs.

This makes sense because most of other symptoms of PPIs are the ones that lead to increased insulin resistance. These can include the growth of pathogenic bacteria, the death of the bacteria that can leave lipopolysaccharides in the system, increased inflammation to all areas of the gut as well as the rest of the body, and a lack of magnesium in the body. These are all large factors when it comes to the development of insulin resistance, and a noticeably big reason why PPI drugs can lead to more permanent diseases that cause greater reflux symptoms.

Other Diseases Associated with PPI Use

The list of diseases doesn't end there. In fact, it is just the beginning. PPI drugs strip the body of electrolytes, vitamins and minerals, increases insulin resistance and wreaks havoc with hormones. This sets the scene for more disease, more pain and a lower quality of life.

The official list of PPI-related diseases include the following:

- Intestinal bacterial Infection
- Malabsorption
- Osteoporosis
- Pneumonia and general ill-health
- Risk of Stomach Cancer
- Risk of Renal Failure
- Cardiovascular Disease
- Stroke
- Dementia

Osteoporosis

A natural follow-on from the mineral deficiencies that we discussed is osteoporosis. PPI drugs tend to cause low calcium levels. Without proper calcium levels, it is unlikely that proper bone formation can occur. In addition to this, insulin resistance prevents bone growth and formation, leaving bones weak and brittle. Since PPI drugs are linked with increased insulin resistance, it is hardly surprising that osteoporosis is one of the most well-known side effects of the drug.

Renal failure

Kidney failure is also linked with PPI use. Kidney failure from PPI use is fairly rare, but how can PPIs cause this? Experts don't have the answers to this yet, but there are some ideas circulating. The kidneys have their own proton pumps, just like the stomach does. Researchers are debating whether PPIs affect the proton pumps that are in the kidneys, but answers have not become available.

Stomach cancer

This seems to be a paradox. Many people begin taking PPIs to reduce the risk of developing esophageal cancer. The downside to PPI treatment is that they leave themselves open to the possibility of developing stomach cancer.

The reason that this occurs is because the stomach works on a feedback system. If acid levels are too low in the stomach, it sends out signals via the hormone gastrin. Gastrin would normally turn the pumps on in the stomach so that the acid levels rise but the drugs have stopped the pumps from working. Since there is still not enough acid in the stomach, the body continues to produce gastrin to correct the imbalance.

High levels of gastrin are known to lead to the development of stomach cancer. PPI doses of 40 to 60mg can produce gastrin levels of up to ten times normal levels. This is known as hypergastrinemia. Some forms of colon cancer are also thought to be related to hypergastrinemia, but there has been no research to link colon cancer to hypergastrinemia from PPI use.

How Much More Can Go Wrong?

Many doctors and scientists argue that PPI drugs could be causing more side effects than are currently recognized. The reason for this is that the drugs have not been extensively studied for particular diseases. So, what further side effects could the drugs be producing?

One suggestion is to compare PPI drugs to the disease atrophic gastritis. Both the drugs and the disease have the same effect on the stomach. They both limit the amount of acid that is produced.

Atrophic Gastritis is a disease of where the cells that produce acid in the stomach start to die off, or simply stop working. It normally causes a decline in stomach acid production as people age. The more that acid production declines, the more symptoms people experience.

Theoretically, the effect of PPIs on stomach acid would be the same as the effect of Atrophic Gastritis. A lot of the diseases that overlap have already been identified.

People with atrophic gastritis are highly likely to develop several serious disorders including these:

- Poor absorption of important vitamins, minerals, and amino acids
- Poor digestion of proteins
- Allergies
- Bronchial asthma in childhood (an obvious exception to "age-related" atrophic gastritis)
- Depression
- Bacterial overgrowth in the stomach and small intestine, leading to symptoms such as heartburn, "gas," constipation, diarrhea, and an increased susceptibility to potentially fatal infections such as cholera and Salmonella
- Pernicious anemia
- Stomach cancer
- Skin diseases, including forms of acne, dermatitis (itching, redness, swelling), eczema, and urticaria (hives)
- Gall bladder disease (gallstones)
- Rheumatoid arthritis
- Lupus erythematosus
- Grave's disease
- Ulcerative colitis

- Chronic hepatitis
- Osteoporosis
- Type 1 (insulin-dependent) diabetes
- Accelerated aging

Notice that many of these are already recognized symptoms of PPI use.

Too dangerous to use?

It is interesting to note that when PPI drugs were newly released onto the market, it was known that they produced gastric cancer in rats. This alarmed some researchers, but supporters of the new drug claimed that this was unique to rats, and that the drugs posed no risk of cancer to humans.

One researcher had this to say, "Until information is available about the effects... the drugs must be categorized as too dangerous to use therapeutically, especially since the proposed therapeutic benefits are minimal." *(Gastroenterol Jpn 1989;24:585- 596)*

These words sound quite prophetic, knowing what we know now. Aside from the possibility to limit development of Barrett's Esophagus, is it wise to use these drugs, when other methods can fix or limit reflux and the pain it causes?

PPI Drugs are Addictive

Giving up PPI drugs can be severe and painful. You may have tried this already and decided to stick to the drugs. You are not alone. Many people have the same experience.

PPI drugs are not addictive in the technical sense of the word, but people cannot just suddenly give up the drugs because the new production of acid causes violent eruptions of reflux episodes. The worst cases of acid reflux often occur after stopping the medication and is commonly called the 'Rebound Effect'.

There are a couple of theories about why the rebound effect occurs.

The first is that the patient on PPI medications becomes sicker over time. That is, the underlying causes of reflux can quietly become worse when PPI drugs are being administered. This has been our main discussion in this chapter, so it is hardly surprising that the effects are worse after stopping the drugs.

The second reason is that PPI drugs affect hormones in the body. During digestion, the body releases a hormone called gastrin to stimulate acid production as mentioned earlier. When PPI drugs are being used, the acid-producing cells fail to work, so the body sends out more gastrin to produce more acid. In a short space of time, there can be exceptionally large amounts of gastrin floating around in the body. For some people, production of high amounts of gastrin becomes the new normal in response to a meal, so when PPI drugs are stopped, the body continues to produce high gastrin levels at mealtimes.

Now that the acid-releasing cells are working, without PPIs, the high levels of gastrin produce extra-high levels of acid that causes some very painful episodes.

This effect normally lasts only a few days. For those that are giving up PPI drugs, those days can be an awfully long and painful experience.

How Long Do PPI Effects Last?

There are many people that ask this question. Usually these are the people that have used the drug for just a couple of weeks and find that they now have bouts of acid reflux that they never had before.

The official line is that the effects of PPIs are meant to last only a few days at the most, but there have been anecdotal reports that some lasted for up to 2 years before acid-producing cells returned to normal.

How to Step Off PPI Drugs Safely

The following points will make the process of quitting PPI drugs easy. Make sure to follow them closely:

- Eat a low carb diet. The lower the carb count the better, and your best options are a ketogenic diet or a zero-carb diet. Also, make sure you are adapted to the new diet before starting to step off the medications.

- Take more magnesium as a supplement. Seek help for this if you have kidney troubles. Kidneys with compromised function cannot excrete magnesium properly. Levels over 350mg per day can cause diarrhea.

- Take a multi-vitamin for good measure. PPI drugs leave your system depleted of vitamins and minerals, and you will need lots of help to improve the situation.

- Follow symptom-lowering actions. Gargle alkaline water between meals, raise bed head, don't eat for at least 3 hours before bed and sleep on your left side. You can find other strategies in the bonus material that comes with this book.

If you are following these guidelines, and you are in ketosis from an extremely low carb diet (or zero-carb diet) it may be possible for you to quit cold-turkey without the usual severe effects.

However, if you want to exercise caution, you can taper the dose down over two or three weeks. You can slowly reduce your dosage in any way that you feel will work for you, but here is an example of one plan that you can consider:

I.   If you are on 40mg twice a day, cut the morning dose in half for 2 or 3 days
II.   Then cut the night dose in half for 2-3 days
III. Cut morning dose in half again, 2-3 days
IV.   Cut night dose in half, 2-3 days

Repeat this until you feel comfortable to replace the PPIs with H2 blockers.

V.   Replace the morning dose with H2 blockers
VI.   Replace the night dose with H2 blockers
VII. Eventually remove the H2 blockers to be antacid-free

Keep the night PPI dose as low as possible. If you have troubles, add H2 blockers to help mitigate the problems.

And one final thought. If you are determined to ensure a pain-free transition off the drugs: try fasting. If you do this, it is important to remember that this can be done *only if you are fully adapted to a ketogenic diet.*

If you want to avoid the rebound effect from excess gastrin at meals, then avoid meals while the drugs are leaving your system over two or three days. Once those days are up, then eat a very small meal at your first meal and increase your portion sizes slowly until you reach your normal meal size.

Conclusion

Congratulations! You have now achieved the biggest two steps in eliminating your reflux: following a low-carb diet and removing acid-suppressors from your system. Your body can begin to recharge and heal. This may take some time and require some lifestyle changes to give it a boost. If you feel up to it, throw in some small, simple hours of fasting, some easy gentle exercise, and some easy stress relief.

At this stage, many people have questions about gut health, stomach health, and whether probiotics are going to help their situation. The answers to these questions are covered in the next few chapters.

Further Information

Several common medications can cause reflux disease and hamper your efforts to eliminate it. The appendix to chapter 4 has a small list of drugs that could be causing your reflux symptoms.

CHAPTER 5

FIX YOUR GUT LINING

The topic of gut health has been attracting a huge amount of interest in the last few years, but I have noticed that many people seem confused about the topic. And rightly so! Science is only just beginning to understand all the intricacies about how our gut system functions and how all the parts link together.

If science is not completely clear on all aspects of gut health, how can we be expected to understand it any better? In the next three chapters we will discuss what we do know about gut health, as well as aspects that are more likely to be rumors.

Intestinal health is often seen as the biggest factor in reflux problems. There are good reasons why people spend so much time trying to fix their gut health. The consequences of poor gut health can be severe.

Gut health is very much tied up with the types of food that we eat, and can lead to diseases such as IBS, IBD, Ulcerative Colitis and Crohn's Disease. Not only can poor gut health be the cause of diabetes, insulin resistance, autoimmunity and food sensitivities, but it can be made worse by those very same diseases.

By now you have started on a diet that will reduce the toxins and bad bacteria in the gut. But diet can go so much further. We will delve into foods for the gut in the chapters on nutrition, but in this chapter, we will focus on the gut itself.

The Gut as an Ecosystem

The gut is like an entire ecosystem. The environment can be healthy, or it can be sick. It is supported and managed by the body, so the way that we eat and live can make a big difference to its health.

Imagine a small forest scene. In a valley, a beautiful stream runs through green pasture, surrounded on both sides by trees. There are fish in the water, birds in the skies, and animals living in the forest. All the creatures are feeding on the grass, eating the leaves and drinking from the water. Some of the animals probably have a symbiotic relationship to one another where they benefit from each other's presence. A bird on a rhino's back is picking off the lice that are trying to infest it. The water is flowing, the breeze is blowing, and the atmosphere is always fresh as it moves through.

There are three important features of this scene that we can relate to the gut.

The first is the terrain. This is the gut lining. Like fertile soil that produces healthy trees and plants, the lining of our gut must be well-formed so that it can produce all the particles that feed and defend the ecosystem within it. An unhealthy gut is like dry, cracked and barren land – it no longer absorbs water or the nutrients that the plants or animals leave behind. It fails to lubricate itself and can't support the balance of life around it. Its usefulness as a barrier between the gut and the body diminishes and grows weaker. Poor health of the gut lining will not only affect the ecosystem within the gut, but the health of all the body, as we will see.

The second is the wildlife. Our gut is inhabited by a broad spectrum of microbes that contribute to the health of the gut lining and to the whole body. Many species of these microbes also support one another, and they all have their places that they live within the gut. Knowing what types of wildlife inhabit your gut may be helpful information but trying to add to it or balance it with probiotics may not create a positive experience, as many people assume. We'll talk about this more.

The third feature is the flow of the environment that keeps everything clean and 'fresh'. A lack of this movement is quite common these days, leading to a stale environment that festers with unwanted creatures, an overgrowth of them, and a build-up of toxic products that linger, without being swept away. This is such an important aspect of gut health that is almost always overlooked, and leads to infestation and overgrowth of pathogenic bugs, much like an unhealthy plague.

But first, let's talk about the terrain, what it looks like, and what can go wrong.

What a Healthy Gut Should Look Like

The gut lining has many roles. The tasks that each gut cell carries out has a role in maintaining both the health of the body and the health of the gut.

The gut is best known for being the part of the body that absorbs nutrients in our food, so that we can live and thrive. The value of this cannot be understated because it is becoming more and more common for people to have nutrient deficiencies when the gut lining is unhealthy. We will find out how this works in a moment.

The gut lining is also a physical barrier that protects us from undigested particles and from pathogens. It is important to keep a good separation between the gut contents and the blood stream on the other side of the gut wall. Particles and pathogens in the gut can create terrible chronic diseases if they were ever able to pass through the gut lining into the bloodstream.

The lining also protects us with immune defenses, by killing and removing pathogens. It has special cells that are dedicated to this task.

And finally, it is thought that the gut that also feeds and supports the bacteria that are most beneficial to us.

There are many more cell types that carry out other tasks for the gut, but these are the main ones that we want to discuss in this chapter. Not only do all the cells work together in harmony, but the terrain of the gut has a special folded formation to increase the effectiveness of what it does.

Let us first look at the types of cells that are in our gut lining, and how they work for our benefit.

Gut Wall Lining

The gut can perform so many functions because it is made up of many different types of cells. Despite their differences, they all join to make up one single united barrier against unwanted particles and organisms. The surprising fact about the gut lining is that the barrier between the gut contents and the bloodstream is only one cell thick.

Cells grow side-by-side along the length of the intestines. The sides of the cells stick together with the help of some special proteins, that help to form this barrier. This link between the cells, formed by the proteins, is known as a tight junction. The tight junctions provide a lot of flexibility, because they are not fixed in place – they can allow the cells to stretch apart, or close back together, if an action of this type is ever called for.

The cells that make up the lining of the gut is always in a state of flux, always changing. This is because cells in the lining only live for a few days, so the entire lining is replaced with new cells every 3 to 7 days. But it is never built the same way. It is always changing according to the greatest needs of the body.

The number of each type of cell varies according to what the body needs at any given time. The body will actually make more of one type if circumstances call for it. So, if you need more help to fight diseases in the gut, the body will make more immune cells in the gut. If organisms are getting through the mucus barrier, or if the mucus lining is getting too thin, the body will make more mucus cells to help build a more stable environment.

Three types of cells are useful to our discussion here, because these are the ones that have the greatest bearing on the factors that can lead to reflux. These are enterocytes, goblet cells and immune cells.

Enterocytes

Enterocytes are the most common type of cell in our intestines, and they absorb the nutrients that we need from our food. The way that they do this is probably not what you would expect. Since there are so many cells lined up side by side, each cell does not have much surface area to absorb nutrients that pass by. Only the tops of the cells are exposed to the gut contents. The Enterocytes get around this problem because of their brush-like appearance at the top of each cell. The brush fibers are called microvilli and they are there to increase the absorptive surface of the cell.

This brush border of the cell also serves another purpose as well. Enterocytes produce their own digestive enzymes known as peptidases and disaccharidases. These enzymes gather in the brush border and break down proteins and sugars from the gut into smaller particles so that they can be absorbed more easily into the cell. Enterocytes also absorb fats, electrolytes, vitamins, minerals, as well as any left-over bile salts that have not attached to fat molecules.

Goblet cells

Goblet cells produce mucus that coats the lining of the intestines. This is simply a gel-like substance that the body produces, and it has quite a number of uses and ways that it protects us.

The first way is by providing simple lubrication to all the cells. Cells are built with a delicate membrane that can be easily damaged. The lack of lubrication would cause rough travelling particles to catch and tear the cell membranes much more easily. And in general, cells of the gut need to live in a moist environment. In the same way, liberal lubrication of the gut allows the easy passage of food through the intestines. Without it, movement of food would be extremely difficult.

Lubrication in this way can probably be described as passive. The mucus is there, and it helps particles to slide past. There is also a much more active way that the body uses mucus. This can be done to move destructive particles, such as fiber, away from the cells.

Actively pushing particles away is the second action that goblet cells use. This is why fiber increases bowel movements. Fiber tears little holes in the cells as it passes by, and the cells react by creating more mucus to push the particles away. The goblet cells also use the same method to keep pathogens away from the intestinal wall and to keep contents in the middle of the gut. In a sense, the goblet cells create a mucus barrier that keeps much of the gut contents separated from the gut wall.

A third way that mucus helps to protect us is by being the carrier of antibodies from the immune system. It would not be helpful to wait until pathogens were attacking the lining of the gut before doing something about it. Instead, the immune system uses mucus to carry out its pre-emptive strikes against pathogens in the gut.

And finally, there has recently been a lot of talk about whether the body also produces mucus to feed microbes that the body wants to support. It has only recently been discovered that some microbes can feed on the mucus along the gut lining, and not just on the undigested fiber particles that we eat. There is still a great deal of speculation about the implications of this, but it may explain why those who eat meat-only diets still seem to sustain healthy populations of gut microbes.

Immune cells

Our body's immune system is also planted right inside the gut. Many of the cells of the gut lining are immune cells, designed to protect us from dangerous bacteria and viruses. In fact, about 70-80% of the body's immune system is located there. This makes sense, because the gut environment is the perfect place for infestation – it is dark, moist and warm.

The immune system in the gut has a couple of tricks it uses to limit or eliminate pathogens that are lurking in the dark.

One method is by heating up the gut wall through inflammation. This can often destroy some of the less harmful and less persistent microbes. This is usually a short-term measure that subsides once the threat has disappeared.

The other method is by having the immune cells produce antibodies. The body doesn't wait for pathogens to arrive at the gut wall before it acts. It has a fairly good idea about what pathogens are out there. It produces antibodies that will target those specific microbes, and it disperses the antibodies out into the gut, via the mucus. Any pathogens that try to move from the food to the gut wall must travel through the mucus where they will be zapped by the antibodies floating around in there.

It is a clever system because it targets that microbes that are harmful and saves the good microbes that the body wants to keep.

Folds of the Gut Lining

One last incredible feature of the intestinal landscape is the way that the intestines are laid out. We have talked about the lining of the gut and the cells that are placed within it. But the gut arranges these parts into one huge landscape within the gut. The reason for the overall structure is to make nutrient absorption more effective.

A normal sized gut can measure anywhere from 5 to 10 meters in length (that's just the small intestines). Normally, this would not be long enough to absorb all the nutrients we need, so the gut fixes this by bunching itself up into folds. This adds more surface area inside the gut. The more surface area we have, the more nutrients we can absorb from our food.

There are three layers of folds in the intestines.

To get a clear picture of this, just imagine one of those very wrinkly dogs – the ones that seem to have too much skin. If you have never seen one, just google 'wrinkly dog'. These dogs have so much skin that it bunches up into waves that roll all the way down its body. If you can imagine this, then you will have a pretty good idea of what the insides of the intestines look like.

These large folds are called Plicae Circulares, and they are the first level of folds in the intestines.

Protruding out from all these larger folds of the intestine, are little finger-like protrusions. This would be like the hair that covers the wrinkly skin on the dogs. In the intestines, these protrusions are about 1mm in length, and they cover the entire surface of the gut, from the beginning to the end. In fact, the definitive identifying feature of the small intestine is whether these hair-like protrusions are present all over the surface. These protrusions are known as villi (singular is called a villus). They increase the surface area even more and they are the second level of folds.

Every single villus in the gut is covered in cells. These cells are the absorbent gut wall lining that is only one single cell thick. Most of these cells are enterocytes, and as we mentioned earlier, every enterocyte cell has the third level of folds. Each cell is covered with its own brush-like surface: many fine projections that are known as microvilli. These microvilli that cover each cell are also particularly important for nutrient absorption.

This arrangement of the cell lining and the folds is very important because many people lose some of the integrity in the lining, and when this happens, many health problems begin to appear. As the lining and the finer, more delicate folds of the intestines are worn away, the protection of the gut lining falters, and every protective feature of the gut that we have described so far is compromised.

What Can Go Wrong?

So far, we have set the scene. Lining all these layers of folds are the cells that do the job of keeping us healthy. The immune system keeps pathogens at bay. The goblet cells produce mucus to keep all the microbes and the food in the middle of the gut, to disperse immune antibodies and to help food pass through the intestines easily. And the enterocytes, of course, are essential to absorbing nutrients. There are many other cells types that work to keep us healthy, and all of them need a healthy gut environment to be able to function properly.

Inflammation

The biggest upset to the function of the intestines is inflammation. And not just any inflammation. A normal inflammatory response to pathogens will last just a short time. Inflammation in the gut becomes dangerous when it lasts for long periods of time, or when it doesn't stop at all. This is known as chronic inflammation.

Chronic inflammation in the intestines normally goes unnoticed. You cannot feel it, but if you are lucky, you may be able to recognize inflammation through symptoms that arise in other areas, such as eczema on the skin. This can give you an indication of what is happening inside your gut.

Inflammation reduces the capacity of your cells to do the jobs that they are designed to do. While inflammation is present, everything changes.

Goblet cells will often begin making more mucus to reduce the 'fire'. This can result in more lubrication and more efficient passage of food through the intestines, but it also means that the enterocytes do not absorb as many nutrients, resulting in nutrient deficiency. With so much mucus keeping everything in the middle of the intestines, there is not much chance for it to absorb through the walls.

In some other scenarios, goblet cells are more likely to dry up, making it difficult for contents to move through efficiently. This can give you the feeling of being 'backed up' or feeling overstuffed even though you may not have eaten for hours.

Excess inflammation can also lead to premature damage and death to cells. This, of course is never a good result. If this type of process continues constantly over a significant period, it can begin to flatten the villi, leading to lowered nutrient absorption.

Another strange consequence of inflammation is a lack of flow in the intestines. This can lead to a build-up of intestinal bacteria, especially in areas where they are not needed or wanted. As the immune system tries to deal with the pathogens, more inflammation is created, making the problem even worse. The pathogens become more prominent in the stagnant contents of the gut.

In addition to this, inflammation creates insulin resistance, as we discussed in the previous chapters. This is particularly important for the gut because continued insulin resistance over very long periods of time can damage the nerves that are needed for gut movement, leading to less movement of gut contents.

Inflammation in the gut is almost always caused by foods – the wrong foods, which is why there are multiple chapters devoted to the topic in book two.

Leaky gut

When inflammation takes hold in the gut, it begins to damage the junctions between the enterocyte cells – those proteins found on the sides of cells that help them to stick together. As these proteins are damaged, the cells begin separating, revealing gaps between the cells.

This condition is known as gut permeability, or more colloquially, as 'Leaky Gut', and indicates a compromised gut barrier where the bloodstream in the body is no longer completely protected from unwanted particles. Various molecules, undigested particles and even pathogens would not normally be able to pass through the gut wall while it is in a healthy state, but when leaks develop between the cells, all of this can change.

This can sound benign at first. After all, the blood stream has its own immune system that it can use to take care of any stray pathogens but this situation can escalate very quickly. The immune system inside the body basically only recognizes two things about particles. It is either food (well-digested food particles), or it is not food (undigested food particles or other particles). And if it is an undigested particle, it must be a pathogen. Bring out the big guns!

In its attempts to rid the bloodstream of perceived pathogens, the body creates a lot more inflammation, and can begin the process of creating antibodies to target the new threat. This is thought to be the most common cause of autoimmune disease, where the body begins destroying its own organs. Autoimmune disease is also a known cause of reflux, but it is so intimately tied up with food intake, that we will be investigating it in the chapters on nutrition. The best course of action at this stage is to focus on healing the gut lining.

Unhealthy or damaged cells

Back in the gut, there is still the possibility that even more damage can be inflicted. In extremely severe cases, where cells are continually bombarded by damaging particles, new cells of the gut fail to be reproduced. Damage can be inflicted by particles such as fiber, plant lectins, oxalates and other toxins that we frequently take in through food. Damage to gut cells can also be accelerated by autoimmune diseases. Whether cell destruction occurs via autoimmune disease or by damaging food particles, it is possible for gut cells to be killed at a higher rate than the body can replace them.

In these cases, the villi that cover the intestines become shorter and shorter. As you can probably guess, those who have this condition are unable to absorb enough nutrients for proper functioning of the body. Not only are the microvilli (the brush-border of each cell) depleting, but entire villi are disappearing as well!

It is good to keep inflammation and other damage under control, because severe inflammation can lead to scarring, and, in very severe cases, to intestinal obstructions.

Take Action to Heal Your Gut

In a normal, healthy person who has no gut trouble at all, the gut has a certain amount of resilience. It can recover from many of the destructive forces that we may throw at it. But in someone who is clearly showing signs of wear and tear from the gut, the healing process has obviously been compromised in some way.

There are two courses of action that you can take. One is to limit the damage, and the other is to actively support your gut's ability to heal.

The first course of action you should take is to stop doing anything that could be causing damage to the gut lining. It would be pointless to embark on a gut-healing protocol if you were continuing to damage your gut at the same time. This would simply keep you sicker for longer.

Most people are unaware how rough foods can be on the lining of the intestines. In a bid to improve their health, many people embark on a health campaign, switching to many fibrous and difficult-to-digest foods. You may have heard some gurus promoting particular foods because they 'scrape the sides of your gut and clean out the debris'. These are definitely the types of foods to avoid.

Also, avoid eating raw vegetables. Vegetables are full of indigestible fiber that can cause micro-tears in the cell walls. They are quite abrasive in the gut. If you want to eat vegetables, choose the non-fibrous parts, and then cook them to break down the cellulose structures to release the nutrients inside. For example, if you are going to have dark leafy greens, cut out and discard the fibrous stem section and then steam the softer leafy sections to break up the remaining indigestible plant structures.

Also, consider eating more animal foods and less plants. This may seem counterintuitive for a number of reasons, but this will all be explained in much more detail in the chapter on nutrition. But, in short, animal products are not fibrous, are completely digestible and all the nutrients are completely bioavailable.

And finally, make sure you are eating foods that are clearly causing no sensitivity issues at all. Any foods that are causing inflammation may be causing other undetected damage too.

The second course of action you should take is to add foods and supplements that are going to support your body's ability to heal.

The primary nutrient that you need to include is fat. Fats are incredibly nourishing for the gut, so if you are already following a well-formed ketogenic diet, then this part should be taken care of already.

Butyric acid is used by the gut lining in the formation of new cells, so it is good to make sure that decent amounts of butyric acid are going to be there for use. In many people, gut bugs can break down indigestible fibers to form butyric acid, but gut bugs can also break down proteins to form butyric acid also. So, if you are eating good quality proteins, then this step should already be underway. If you want to try supplementing, there are capsules you can take to transport butyric acid into your intestines. Products such as butter contain high amounts of butyric acid, but most of it is broken up through digestion in the stomach.

L-Glutamine is an amino acid that is a great energy source for immune and intestinal cells. It is the most abundant amino acid in our bodies, but it is still often taken as a supplement to support the gut, by its action in maintaining the integrity of the intestinal wall. This amino acid heals all tissue in the body and helps those with irritated tissue in the digestive tract. In addition to this, it is known as the calming amino acid, and is somewhat effective at reducing anxiety.

If you are eating a diet comprised mostly of animal products, you are more than likely getting a good dose of l-glutamine, but feel free to experiment with supplements if you believe they could assist you further.

Calcium is useful in healing leaky gut. At this stage, it is probably best taken as a supplement. Since you probably want to take it in doses that are higher than normal, you won't find these levels in animal foods, except dairy which you should be excluding at the moment. And the plant sources of calcium are accompanied by some nasty particles that we will discuss in the chapters on nutrition.

If you are supplementing with calcium, then you should probably also be taking vitamin K2. K2 is available only in grass-fed animal products, and not in plants. It is possible for the body to convert plant-based K1 into the useable K2, but this is not a reliable way to maintain the health that you are looking for. After all, if you are deficient in any vitamins and minerals needed for the conversion process, then the plan will fail. Animal foods from grass-fed animals that contain fats such as eggs and butter should be abundant in this vitamin.

And lastly, a note about vitamin K2. This nutrient has only become the subject of popular discussion recently, so it is not usually seen recommended in conventional medical recommendations. Vitamin K has numerous benefits to your body and to your gut. Even though your liver stores a certain level of vitamin K for use by the body, there are even higher amounts found in other organs. The salivary glands have 190 times more than the liver. The brain contains 290 times more. And the pancreas contains 1870 times more.

For this reason, researchers believe that K2 may be involved in maintaining calcium in teeth and bones and regulating the microbiome in the mouth. In the brain it is involved in the synthesis of cells and helps with nerve function, cognitive function, memory, and neurological diseases. And in the pancreas, with such high levels, many believe it must play a substantial role in regulating blood glucose levels. All these organs are involved in maintaining gut health.

In the gut, the pancreas secretes large amounts of vitamin K2. K may increase the effectiveness of the intestinal mucus by balancing pH, blocking inflammation, sealing up leaky gut and ridding the body of toxins. It also assists other components of the gut that play a role in decreasing inflammation and eliminating toxins effectively.

Most people who have heard about K2 know it for its action on fighting atherosclerotic plaques and calcium deposits in arteries that lead to heart disease. That was the original reason that I began including high amounts of grass-fed butter to my foods. That alone could be reason enough, but with a profile like this, K2 is something that you should be including in your diet if you want to fix your gut and overcome reflux disease.

Note: Some natural food components such as vitamin K and other foods such as fish oils can have a thinning effect on the blood. Take care with this if you are already on blood-thinning medications. Always inform your doctor of any dietary changes you are making.

How to Support the Gut Lining

Nutrient support

- Butyric acid found in butter is food for gut cells
- Take L-Glutamine to help heal the gut lining
- Calcium can help to heal leaky gut
- Vitamin K2 to accompany Calcium, and heal leaky gut, to reduce insulin resistance, and regulate bile production

Foods

- Eat foods that are not rough on the lining
- Protein foods can break down to produce butyric acid in the gut
- Grass-fed animal foods contain vitamin K2 in the fats
- Cook all vegetables. Raw vegetables can be abrasive to the gut lining
- Avoid undigestible or abrasive supplements such as fiber
- Eat foods that do not trigger food sensitivities

Other

- Avoid aspirin and other painkillers as they shrink the mucosal layer protecting the gut lining, the stomach lining and the esophagus lining, leaving them all open to greater damage.

Further Reading

- *Vitamin K in Health and Disease* by John W Suttie
- *Fiber Menace* by Konstantin Monastyrsky

CHAPTER 6

UNDERSTANDING GUT BACTERIA

The second section of the gut that we need to discuss is its inhabitants. There is a symbiotic relationship between the wildlife and its habitat. In our world, the land provides grasses and plants for the animals to graze on, and in turn the animals break up the soil and fertilize it to make the soil ripe for new growth. In the same way, the bacteria in our gut feed on whatever we provide for them, but in turn they provide nutrients that support the function of our bodily systems.

The relationship between us and our gut bacteria goes far beyond just receiving a few nutrients. Most people realize that the gut microbiome is an important part of battling reflux, but many people think that we can live a lifestyle that destroys many of the bacterial species, and then replace microbes in the gut with a few supplements. This is not the case.

Having a healthy gut relies on preserving the original inhabitants of your gut as much as possible. There has been a trend over the last few decades that has seen increased use of antibiotics in allopathic medicine, as well as anti-fungal and anti-bacterial products in the natural medicines. These treatments will change your gut and your overall health permanently, and unless you are willing to undergo a fecal transplant to renew the diversity of your gut microbiome, you are unlikely to recover from the destructive practices that we have all been subject to.

If you are having difficulties with the bacteria in your gut, if you are overcome with bloating and all types of intestinal discomforts, it may be tempting to take the easy route to fix it. This rarely works effectively, and there are much more effective ways that we will discuss in this chapter and the next.

Use of Antibiotics

One of the greatest tragedies of our modern times is the overuse, and inappropriate use of antibiotics. The fact is that this practice is making us sicker, not healthier, and antibiotics should only be used in serious medical cases. Up until now, it has been assumed that antibiotics are perfectly safe to use at any time, and it is only very recently that evidence to the contrary has surfaced.

We gain our bacterial populations from our parents, siblings and close contacts. Microbes have been found to affect our health in many ways – you can probably see trends in amongst family members. Some bacteria change our height, our weight, our immune function and they protect us from diseases. Other bacteria break down the indigestible parts of our diets.

This may sound familiar, or even obvious, but we don't know all these facts because we have studied the bacteria themselves. Much of what we know comes from comparing people who have taken antibiotics with those that haven't. Some studies, and even some unfortunate historical events, have allowed researchers to observe the differences between the two groups of people.

Some of the chronic diseases that are gripping us in our modern era are the result of the antibiotics we have taken over the course of our lifetimes.

For example, why is weight gain such a problem? Studies have shown that those that take antibiotics are more likely to put on weight. Another factor that affects this is the age that you start on antibiotics. When antibiotics are taken early in life, the effects of weight gain become permanent. This is probably a major reason why the world is becoming fatter. Babies are increasingly being given antibiotic treatments incredibly early on in life. In some countries it is built into the health plan for every child.

Antibiotics also leave us open to greater infection. They remove the protection offered by the resident microbes against any invading microbes. Remember this if you are ever travelling to poorer areas of the world. If you take antibiotics before or during the trip, you leave yourself particularly vulnerable to infection for at least a month afterward. This can increase your chances of getting infected, as well as having a much more severe reaction to pathogens than you would have had without prior antibiotic treatment.

In addition to this, it has been found that the development of Intestinal Bowel Disease, such as Crohn's or Ulcerative Colitis, is usually preceded by a course of antibiotic treatment. Taking antibiotics can triple your risk of developing Crohn's disease, and the more antibiotics that you take, the higher the risk becomes, at around 18% higher risk for every course of antibiotics!

It also has a great impact on autoimmune diseases. Studies have found that at the time that people are diagnosed with celiac disease, antibiotics were 40% more likely to have been prescribed in the preceding months. H.Pylori is one of the microbes responsible for preventing celiac disease. Another autoimmune disease, Type 1 diabetes, is accelerated by taking antibiotics early in life, and has already become an epidemic with children developing the disease at younger and younger ages.

I might also draw your attention to an interesting fact about C-section births. This is not about antibiotics, but it shows what a lack of microbes can do, because a natural birth, which is very messy, involves a transfer of microbes from the mother to the child. Studies are showing that babies born via C-Section method are at increased risk of becoming obese and developing asthma, allergies and autoimmune diseases as they grow up. The theory behind this is that the newborn babies have not been exposed to all the microbes that they would in a natural birth. Since this information has become more widespread, some doctors take the time to ensure that microbial populations from the vagina are transferred to the baby immediately after birth to reduce the likelihood of future diseases.

The list of diseases affected by antibiotics goes on. Eczema, dermatitis and hay fever associated with asthma. Allergies, such as those to peanuts, are also becoming increasingly common. Conditions of brain development that lead to autism are also thought to be affected by a loss of microbes very early in life.

Groups of scientists are now becoming concerned about the risk posed by antibiotics for future generations. The micro-world is something that we still do not know much about, but we are still ploughing ahead, eliminating as many as we can with all our antibacterial products. We know that bacteria such as H.Pylori are dying out, and these have been with us for thousands of years. How many other ancient microbial species are we eliminating? And how many have we brought to extinction already?

Will probiotics help?

Many people are led to believe that taking antibiotics is ok, because afterward we can simply take some probiotics to make up for the loss. Unfortunately, it does not work this way.

For one thing, probiotics are collections of luminal microbes. These are the ones that munch on the fiber that we eat. And for another thing, there is no probiotic that replaces the gut wall microbes that support our immune system. Once those ones are lost, there is no turning back. We'll discuss these two types of microbes in a moment.

As for the luminal microbes, think of it this way. A healthy gut can have hundreds of different microbes residing there. Let's say there are 500 different species and strains. After a course of antibiotics, let's say that 300 of them are wiped out. Some studies have shown greater losses, but for the sake of our example here, 300 species is a great loss. So, now there are only 200 different types left.

A bottle of probiotics at the shop only has about 10 different types of probiotics in it. That can bring the total back up to 210 bacterial types, but what about the other 290? These are now lost, and all the benefits that they provided are now gone too. And you will never know what benefits they were providing to you.

The only thing that you will know is that as you get older, more and more diseases begin to develop. You can reflect and speculate about whether the diseases that you developed in the past developed soon after a course of antibiotics. And all the other diseases that have been developing since then, were they the result of bacterial loss as well? You will probably never find out.

Now that we know that antibiotics, and microbe loss is associated with so many diseases, it is difficult to know which ones are developing because of old age, and which ones are a result of our poor lifestyle decisions. The best course of action you can take for your gut health is to conserve your own gut bacteria as much as possible, because no one has any idea how changes can affect you.

How Much Do We Really Know?

Our knowledge of the microbiome is in its infancy. Study on the microbiome has only just begun. The old-fashioned idea that all microbes are best destroyed has finally passed, for the most part, and scientists are beginning to discover all the ways that microbes can benefit our health.

Some exciting discoveries have been made, but the information that we have discovered so far is very limited.

We know that there is a symbiotic relationship between us and our microbes. They need us for survival, and it is becoming apparent that we also need them for our own survival. We need them for the biproducts that they create, and for the way that they train and maintain our immune systems to keep us healthy.

There are at least 2 layers of microbes in the gut: the ones that attach themselves to the gut wall and the 'Luminal' microbes that feed on the food in the middle of the intestines. These two layers of microbes are separated by a layer of mucus that lines the intestinal walls. The wall-hugging microbes are protected under the layer of mucus, and the other luminal microbes occupy all the rest of the space in the middle of the gut.

Luminal microbes

Luminal microbes are the ones that have caught the interest of most studies. These are the ones that show up in stool tests because they are the ones that feed on the indigestible fibers in our diets. They break down the fibers and produce a number of products such as butyric acid which help to keep our gut cells nourished and healthy. They also create many other products that our bodies absorb such as B-vitamins, or other types of nourishment for cells.

But the world of 'good' bacteria is not all rosy. Many microbes that find their way into the gut create awful gases and other substances that smell rotten. I know this because there was a long time that I was not able to eat onions or eggs without regretting the odor later. Although this can be annoying, it is usually fairly harmless. These bacteria can show up in stool tests as either good or benign.

In addition to this, there can also be many microbes that really are harmful. The body's immune system takes steps to remove these, but it can often be unsuccessfully achieved.

This is a situation that I found myself in after drinking some 'undrinkable' water at a campsite many years ago. I was left with dysentery for many years, until I was able to clear it all up with one of the diets listed in the previous chapters.

Many people believe that long-term dysentery and intestinal bacterial problems are reserved for Third World countries where conditions are unsanitary, but that is not the case. More people in the Western world are experiencing bacterial overgrowth, for different reasons, and are not finding solutions with antibiotics, whether natural or pharmaceutical. The only solution that worked for me was the combination of steps that I am revealing in this book.

These steps work to limit pathogenic bacteria, support good bacteria and work with the gut's own in-built cleansing processes, which we will talk about in the next chapter.

For me, these steps had a great impact on the luminal bacteria of my gut, and eliminated those microbes that like to produce sulphurous and other smelly gases.

Science knows a lot more about the luminal microbes than the wall-layer microbes. A large number of luminal microbes have been studied, and we continue to learn about their benefits, as well as their drawbacks. These days it is even possible to obtain detailed stool tests that identify the various populations, and determine which ones are considered good, harmful or neutral to your health.

How do we know whether each of these strains are good or not? The opinions drawn in conclusions of studies are never set in stone. It seems that opinion about the usefulness of each strain swings back and forth as studies continue to identify the good and bad points of each one.

For this reason, don't be too swayed by the opinions of others. The luminal microbes are important, but in many cases, it is debatable as to which bugs and how many of them we really need.

Out of the two layers of gut microbes, the luminal bugs are probably the less important microbes in many ways. After all, these are the bugs that are naturally transitory. They don't set up shop the way other gut bugs do. They enter the system, they party, and then they leave. Some will stick around if we eat enough of the foods that will keep them there, and the body even has its own tricks to support the gut bugs that it wants to keep there.

Despite all the good that they do for us, it is the set of microbes at the wall layer that can have a much greater impact on our health. These also tend to be the ones that are irreplaceable once they are lost.

Wall-layer microbes

The wall-layer microbes can have an enormous impact on our health because they interact directly with us to manipulate body systems or the immune system. They teach us which microbes are harmful to us and prompt the immune system to create antibodies against them. 80% of our immune system sits in the lining of the gut, and these microbes help us to make good use of it.

Unfortunately, despite the enormous impact they can have on our health, there have been very few studies conducted to understand them. We know truly little about the wall-side microbes and how they manipulate bodily systems. We don't even know which species tend to inhabit our systems.

You may never find out which ones are living inside your body, because they rarely come out in stool tests. They tend to cling to the gut wall as everything else slides past them toward the exit.

There are a few researchers that have voiced concerns about our lack of knowledge of these microbes. There is some concern that some species that have inhabited the human intestines for thousands of years, the ones that have been protecting us from chronic diseases are becoming extinct. We may be eradicating important ancient species with antibiotics, without ever having discovered them!

While luminal microbes can produce some butyric acid to nourish cells, and some enzymes that help with various processes, the gut-wall microbes may be protecting us from autoimmune diseases, asthma, acid reflux, Barrett's Esophagus, and many other serious diseases.

You may be surprised to learn that one of these ancient microbes is Helicobacter Pylori.

H. Pylori

H. Pylori has been seen as the cause of stomach ulcers and stomach cancer in recent decades. It wasn't too long ago that the mantra was 'A good H. Pylori is a dead H. Pyori'.

Martin Blaser, author of Missing Microbes, has spent the last forty years studying this particular microbe, and although his early research drew the links between H. Pylori and stomach cancer, his later research revealed that there is a lot more to the story. It is not a simple case of bacteria plus stomach equals cancer. For one thing, you must be supplied with these bacteria at birth, so that it can adjust to its host. It is a very intimate relationship, and if you pick it up later in life, the relationship just does not work out.

H. Pylori has been in decline in populations of the western world for the last 100 years. The evidence that we have on hand reveals that 150 years ago, most people carried H. Pylori in their systems. The more developed we have become, the faster it has declined. Blaser's research revealed that while the bacteria were declining, many diseases have been rising, quite sharply.

His research was the first to reveal that H. Pylori had a protective effect against GERD and associated diseases such as Barrett's esophagus, and asthma. Without H. Pylori, a person is up to eight times more likely to develop GERD. As a result, it also gave protection against esophageal diseases that are normally associated with GERD.

Lately, a general theory has developed linking GERD with asthma. The idea is that acid reflux gets into the airways, irritates that lining of the airways and causes asthma. Blaser showed that H.Pylori protects against asthma, whether the patient has GERD or not, and posed the question: Does acid reflux really cause asthma, or are the two diseases simply caused by a lack of H.Pylori?

As it turns out, H.Pylori builds up the body's resistance to allergens, and increases people's ability to turn off an allergic response. In fact, those with H.Pylori tend to grow more immune system cells that are associated with regulating immune responses. The immune system, like most systems, needs to have checks and balances so that the active part of it does not tear the body apart in its attempt to wage war against pathogens. It just so happens that H.Pylori upregulates and trains the system to calm itself, and not get too excited over every little thing that turns up.

This means, that an immune system without regulation can result in problems with histamine intolerance, or any other intolerance, or even autoimmune disease.

Unfortunately the use of antibiotic treatments can destroy H.Pylori populations very easily, eliminating them altogether. This can have consequences on health, leaving people susceptible to developing intolerances and autoimmune diseases.

Discovering this research was interesting, because it also follows the development of my own acid reflux condition. After I developed a severe case of dysbiosis in 2000, I was given several antibiotic courses over the next few years, to try to improve the situation. I began having troubles with my voice, and I was officially diagnosed with reflux around 2004. I was never tested for H.Pylori at the time, so unfortunately I will never know if H.Pylori was responsible for the good health I had prior to the antibiotic treatments.

If you find that you have a case of H.Pylori, think carefully about whether to eradicate it or not. The conventional advice will always say to remove it, but if you have had it since birth, it may be protecting you from many different diseases. Either way, there are positive and negative points to having H.Pylori in your gut. You may want to investigate what other factors are causing your reflux first before going ahead and removing the specific bacteria that may be offering a certain measure of protection from many chronic diseases.

How effective are probiotics?

Many people try to improve their gut health by taking probiotics. There is nothing wrong with this, but keep in mind that probiotics do not help everybody. I mention this because the prevailing information on this topic says that you must, must, absolutely must take probiotics to maintain optimal health. This is simply not true. They never seemed to help me – I was more likely to experience a negative reaction – and they may not help you either.

Although probiotics are good, there are situations where taking probiotics will make your symptoms worse. And besides, your body can probably deal with the situation itself. I'll talk about how it can do that in a moment.

For a third of people who take them, probiotics provide a good result. For another third there is no noticeable response, and the final

30% of people actually experience a bad reaction. This is most often due to the development of histamines.

When it comes to cases of bacterial overgrowth in the gut, such as SIBO or Candida, probiotics are of dubious value, and there are better ways to deal with this situation.

Having said that, some people do find that probiotics help with some conditions. It is worth experimenting with probiotics, and if you are not experiencing any negative reactions, then there may be no reason to avoid them. Just make sure to avoid probiotics that are mixed up in dairy, such as kefir and yogurt, and the ones made with grains.

Popular Theories

Personally, I don't subscribe to many of the popularized assumptions about gut health. There are just so many things that we don't know about the microbiome. And there are so many recommendations that exacerbate the negative gut symptoms.

I also don't agree with the idea of 'farming' our gut bugs with high volumes of fiber and lots of different types of plants to attract lots of different types of microbes. The problem is that this style of eating can promote a lot of digestive complaints. Wind, GERD, heartburn, stomach pain, constipation. Is all this pain worth following some untested science?

For one thing, we don't really know what drives gut diversity. The numbers can grow and diminish without any help from us, but what is the cause? Does low diversity of the microbiome cause disease? Or does disease cause low diversity? No one knows for sure, but there is some evidence that it is disease that affects the microbe populations.

There is a new theory that suggests that our bodies feed microbes with the mucus that we produce. This would make sense because the digestive tract produces different types of mucus at different sections of the gut. And at each of these sections, the microbe colonies also differ, so keeping them fed with different types of mucus could make sense. Presumably, the body does this because these are the microbes that it wants to support. And good support could mean good diversity.

Overall, the best steps you can take for your microbiome is to simply avoid foods and supplements that will destroy them. If you ever become ill, try to avoid taking antibiotics unless necessary. And let the microbes take care of themselves. A healthy body supports a healthy microbiome. Your body, it seems, can support them simply fine without much extra input from you.

Some Pointers for a Healthy Microbiome

- Make sure food is well digested (stay clear of antacids, PPIs and other things that hamper digestive capacity).

- Avoid Antibiotics, anti-bacterials and anti-fungal treatments.

- Avoid indigestible foods and supplements. Eat more foods that are completely digestible.

- Stay on a low carb diet. Keep the carb count as low as you can.

- Feel free to take probiotics if they do not cause negative reactions.

- Avoid probiotic and fermented products for now, especially those made from dairy or grains.

- Consider taking N-Acetylcysteine (NAC) to break up biofilms. This can allow the immune system to reach pathogens that are hiding amongst intestinal folds. Short-term use only.

Further Reading

- *Missing Microbes* by Martin Blaser

CHAPTER 7

HOUSEKEEPER OF THE INTESTINES

Of all the places in our bodies, the intestine is the organ most likely to be unclean. Food particles tend to get caught up in all the folds of the intestines and amongst the villi, as the rest of the food moves through. Does all this food and debris just sit there and fester until the next wave of food moves through? Absolutely not!

When we were comparing the gut environment to a countryside scene, we mentioned the flowing rivers and breezes that move everything along, so that the area remains clean, fresh and sanitary. When you imagine the inside of your gut, the image that comes to mind might not quite be flowing rivers and fresh breezes, but I'm sure I don't need to ask if you would prefer your gut to be a clean and healthy environment. The gut has a process that does just that!

The small intestines have an automated process called the Migrating Motor Complex (MMC), and this is something that you are really going to want to know about. In fact, when I first learned about the MMC, it was another one of my 'bowl-me-over' moments. I had never heard it mentioned anywhere in acid-reflux circles, and even now it doesn't get a lot of discussion.

The MMC has the potential to cure people of IBS, IBD, SIBO, Candida, as well as Crohn's disease and leaky gut and a host of other intestinal problems that involve infections and inflammation. A potential cure!

In fact, the words "potential cure" probably sounds a bit over the top. So, let me re-phrase that. The MMC can be switched on or switched off, and the biggest problem is that most people have it switched off for most of the time.

When the MMC is switched off, there is no clean-up after food, and the intestines become a playground for bacteria, yeasts and pathogens of all sorts. It allows the inhabitants of the lower intestines to migrate up into the small intestines where they are not supposed to be. The bacteria can begin to build biofilms between the folds of the intestines and take up permanent residence there. This is when intestinal infections begin to take hold.

But why would the MMC be switched off? You may be surprised to find out that eating habits are to blame. And more surprisingly, some very common reflux advice could be doing the same!

What is the MMC?

The MMC is a highly active process of the intestinal system. As the "Housekeeper of the Intestines", its role is to make sure that everything is clean and sanitary, to avoid unnecessary outbreaks of infection or inflammation.

The MMC is all about motility. But there is a little more to motility than just cleanliness. Motility also takes care of digestion. We'll talk about digestion in the next chapter. Cleanliness and digestion are two very different actions in the gut, but they are two sides of the same coin. They go hand-in-hand. It is a little like preparing meals in the kitchen. Cooking involves making a mess in the kitchen. And after you are done with the meal, you clean everything up. The intestines are just like this when you eat. Digestion makes a mess, and then afterward it needs to be cleaned up.

Before going on, it is important to note that gut motility is not about 'bowel movements'. Bowel movements take place in the large intestine, but in this section, we will focus on the gut movements that only take place in the small intestine (and the stomach). These types of motions are essential to health, but they go completely unnoticed, so you would not even know about them unless you were told about them.

In this action, one great sweep is executed from the stomach, through all 10 meters of small intestines, all the way down to the lower intestines. There is no churning or mixing involved. The purpose is simply to move contents along.

This sweeping action cleans up any left-over particles that have been left behind during the digestive process, as well as any intestinal cells from the gut wall that have died. Left-over particles are only going to be a harbor for pathogens and overgrowth of any other microbes. The small intestines tend to house very few microbes, so this action ensures that the presence of bacteria remains minimal.

And just like a real live housekeeper, the intestines also have their own disinfectants as well. To aid in the cleaning action, a small amount of enzyme and bile solution is released from the pancreas and gallbladder to help disinfect the area from pathogens. The MMC has a particular reputation for keeping pathogens out of the system.

This action of the MMC usually happens when you are no longer actively digesting food because this is the clean-up and sanitization process. It has a particular timing to it, as well as its own set of rules, so if you want your system to function at its peak, then you will need to play the rules of the game.

Fortunately, there are not too many rules, but most people do not know them or follow them. In fact, the only real rule is to leave adequate time in between meals.

Rules of the MMC

An important feature of the MMC is that it works to a clock. It starts up a few hours after the previous meal, and then repeats the action periodically, about once every 90 - 120 minutes (or up to 4 hours in some individuals).

The strength and effectiveness of the sweeps depend on a few factors, but ideally, they begin in the stomach and continue all the way to the end of the intestines. When the conditions are not quite right, or a part of the system is not working well, the sweeps may be shorter and less effective.

Typical MMC cycle

MMC begins around 3 hours after your last meal.

It has 4 phases:

I.   Phase 1 – Quiet phase with no contractions (approx. 45-60 mins)

II.   Phase II – Low motor activity with randomly timed contractions (approx. 25 mins)

III.   Phase III – Fast, strong and evenly spaced waves of contractions (5-15 mins)

IV.   Phase IV – Rapid decrease of contractions (approx. 15 mins)

The whole cycle takes 1.5 to 2 hours to complete.

During phase 1, the gallbladder refills itself with bile collected from the liver. Prior to this stage the gallbladder would have been emptied from the previous meal.

Just before phase 3 begins, the gallbladder empties the bile into the duodenum. Phase 3 will begin as soon as bile is detected inside the duodenum. If everything is working well, this will be a slow, even release from the gallbladder. The gallbladder then begins the process of refilling itself with bile from the liver and continues to do so until the body is ready for phase 3 of the next MMC cycle.

During phase 3, contractions in the stomach deposits acidic gastric juices into the duodenum. Bicarbonate is secreted from the pancreas to neutralize the acid. During this process, some of the bicarbonate backs up into the stomach, which helps to restore a resting pH.

Peristaltic waves from the MMC sweep the bile and the gastric juices through the gut. Bile is antibacterial and it carries out its special task of killing unwanted bacteria.

When the bile acids reach the last section of the small intestines, the ileum, they bind to receptors so that the bile can be reabsorbed into the body for recycling. At the same time, the same receptors release antimicrobial peptides that help to keep all types of microbes (good or bad) in low proportions. This prevents overgrowth of any bacteria, good or bad.

In this way, the bile is preserved and is reused for further digestion and cleaning cycles. In fact, science has not confirmed what initiates the MMC cycles, but one theory suggests that the recycling of bile, along with the filling and emptying of the gallbladder has a major role in it.

All about bile

Your body tends not to discard bile that it makes but aims to reuse it instead. Bile continues to circulate in and out of your digestive system throughout the day. This is known as enterohepatic circulation.

Here's the way that it works. Bile is normally stored in the gallbladder and is secreted from the gallbladder during digestion of a meal, or during the cycles of the MMC. As it travels through the small intestines almost all of it is reabsorbed back into the body. It travels through the bloodstream to the liver where it is sent back to the gallbladder for storage. And the cycle repeats itself.

Bile acids can circulate through this same course 7-10 times a day. Over the course of a day only 5% of all the bile is lost in feces.

One use that the body has for bile is detoxification. Toxins, such as LPS can trigger harmful immune responses, but bile can safely capture LPS, after which it is sent to the liver for processing, and then sent back into the intestines for excretion. The other important use for bile acids is as an antimicrobial agent. The presence of bile tends to keep the numbers of pathogenic bacteria low in the small intestines, but at the same time it supports our friendly bacteria.

Various friendly bacteria, such as lactobacilli and bifidobacteria, have evolved with humans for thousands of years, and have developed traits that allow them to colonize our gut. They are bile-resistant. This is great because it gives them a distinct advantage against pathogens.

With this resistance to bile, there is now the danger that these friendly bacteria have the capacity to become overgrown in the intestines. But the body has an answer for this too.

As all the contents move into the last section of the intestines (the ileum), receptors in the ileum bind to the bile, and transport it into the bloodstream. The reception of bile also causes a secretion of some antimicrobial peptides into the intestines. These antimicrobial particles act on all the bacteria, both the good ones and the bad ones, to keep total numbers to a minimum.

This is especially important in the ileum because all types of bacteria can escape from the large intestine and move up into this section of the small intestines. The showering of antimicrobial particles in this section, as well as the bile that travels through here, can keep harmful bacteria at bay.

And finally, in addition to all of this, bile also maintains the tight junctions in the gut wall of the small intestines, so that they stay closed. In other words, it combats leaky gut by decreasing intestinal permeability. This is especially useful while it is cleaning the gut, to ensure loose particles and bacteria have no way to slip across the barrier.

If we allow our gut system to sweep through with bile multiple times a day, then we could keep our intestines free from harmful bacteria and toxins and have a way to mend a leaky gut wall. This sounds easy, and it is, but there are still a few things that we need to know.

Strength and length of MMC movement

There are times and situations when the MMC will not work quite so well. A strong sweep of the gut will start from the stomach and end where the ileum finishes. Weaker sweeps may start in the duo-denum and only make it part way to the end.

In order to maintain the best and strongest sweeps of the intes-tines, the vagus nerve needs to be stimulated. This nerve travels from the brain and connects to all the organs of the gut. This same nerve heightens your sense of relaxation, raises your sense of smell and taste, and increases your stomach's digestive capacity.

When your mind is calm and you are feeling happy, the vagus nerve is fully activated, and the MMC works at its best. At these times, contractions begin in the stomach and travel the full length of the small intestines, to the end of the ileum.

On the other hand, the antagonist to vagus stimulation is stress. Stress puts a damper on the vagus nerve, so the MMC is no longer regulated by vagus nerve activation. The MMC action still goes ahead, but over a shorter length of the intestines and with less strength. The action begins in the duodenum, not the stomach, and may not even reach the ileum, where a lot of the disinfecting action happens. In addition to this, the gastric juices from the stomach and pancreas won't be included, and the gallbladder will release less bile. This can eventually become a disaster if you are prone to developing microbial infections or overgrowth in your system.

The MMC is even weaker at night. When sleeping, the MMC still works, but it is much more subdued and not as effective at clean-ing. It is best not to rely on night-time cycles for intestinal clean-ing. They do not cover the entire intestinal tract from the stomach to the ileum, so the best course of action would be to encourage MMC cycles to run throughout the day.

How to Switch the MMC On

The important fact about the MMC is that it stops as soon as food is consumed. A meal of 450 calories is enough to switch it off for the next 3 hours. Stretching the stomach by consuming food tends to interrupt the MMC, and any hormones related to digestion are prone to override anything else that is helping the MMC to work.

How much can you eat without interrupting the MMC? Small snacks and drinks can sometimes be consumed with only a little pause to the MMC timing. The number of calories included in the snack can make a difference to how long the MMC is interrupted, and the types of calories make a difference too. Fats cause the longest disruption to the process, with carbohydrates causing a shorter disruption, and protein causing the least.

Most of the world keeps up a routine that does not allow for MMC function. For example, if your first meal of the day is at 8am, then the MMC is due to kick in after about 3 or 4 hours. But instead, most people will eat at around 10:30, just two and a half hours later. And then the next meal will be 2 or 2.5 hours after that. Afternoon tea is usually about the same time later, and then dinner will probably be timed just as the MMC is due to start up.

So, for most of the day, the cleaning action of the intestines is switched off, and only has a chance to work overnight while you are meant to be sleeping. This can greatly increase the chances of bacterial overgrowth during the day, and a night-time clean up may not be enough to clear the damage.

Frequent small meals (again!)

One of the worst pieces of advice I have ever heard given to reflux patients is to eat frequent small meals. This is usually about 6 small meals spread evenly over the course of the day. The theory behind the small meals comes from an attempt to reduce the amount of food sitting in the stomach at any given time. This makes sense, because if there is something wrong with your digestive action, then a larger load of food is more likely to result in reflux. This allows digestion to have its time but cuts out on the MMC. MMC needs to have its time, too. It really should not be a choice of one of these over the other.

Following the advice of small frequent meals means that the intestines are rarely given the chance to be cleaned up. There is more room for pathogens to take hold in the debris and for inflammation to become an issue. Irritable bowel syndrome and Small Intestinal Bacterial Overgrowth (SIBO) are known to be issues in people with limited or incomplete MMC movements. And as we know, inflammation and bacterial overgrowth are more likely to cause all the problems that lead to increased reflux, including insulin resistance.

Eating small frequent meals could be a disaster for health, and if you have been following this diet style, I would suggest that you consider changing your habits. If you really must focus on small meals, you can find out more about how to do this more effectively in the chapters on Nutrition.

How to time your meals

The best way to activate the MMC is to space out your meals. What we are looking for in the MMC cycle are the phase 3 contractions. These are the ones that do the bulk of the work. They happen right at the end of the MMC cycle, so we need to make sure that the full cycle is occurring before we can get the full benefit.

Remember that the MMC cycles begin at least 3 hours after finishing a meal and lasts for almost 2 hours. This means that we will need to wait at least 5 hours between meals, in order to get the benefit of just one MMC cycle. Ideally, we would get 2 cycles in before we had the next meal. That would be 7 hours between meals. So, what would this look like, in terms of meal timing?

There are a few choices.

Wake in the morning and eat. If you wake at 6 am, and you eat, then the next meal of the day would not be until 1pm. And the third meal of the day would be at 8pm.

These timings might not be very practical for most people. For one thing, many people may not wake that early in the morning, which would put the timings out for the rest of the day. A second reason is that the last meal of the day does not leave enough time for full digestion before going to sleep.

Daily fasting to optimize the MMC

A better way to approach gut health would be to incorporate fasting into a daily routine. This is extremely easy to do, and most people have no trouble carrying it out because you can still eat your full count of calories every day.

The most popular style for this is the 16/8 method. This is where you restrict your hours of eating to one 8-hour window of time every day. For example, you can skip breakfast in the morning and have your first meal at 12pm and your last meal at 7pm or 8pm.

With this fasting method, your body's daytime routine might look a little like this:

- 6am-12pm: 3 cycles of MMC
- 12pm-3pm Digesting midday meal
- 3pm-7pm – 2 cycles of MMC
- 10pm-6am Sleep

This routine would allow 5 cycles of MMC action throughout the day! Of course, many people eat more during their 8-hour feeding window. This would reduce the number of active MMC cycles, but if you want to optimize your health, eating less often would be the best option.

Another version of this diet is known as OMAD, or one-meal-a-day. This is also becoming immensely popular in a lot of health circles and allows the greatest amount of time for your gut to clean and heal.

Combining fasting options

Combining a daily fasting routine with some extra, more traditional-style fasting options could give a boost to your intestinal health as well as your overall wellbeing. This is easiest to do once the daily fasting routine becomes your normal eating routine.

The best way would be to add one or two days of water-fasting, every week or 2 to really clean out your system. One or 2 days of fasting is very safe and is actually very popular in the modified version of fasting called the 5/2 diet strategy.

It is possible to transition to 1 and 2 day fasts from your normal eating routine. One option could simply be to lengthen your time between meals. If you are normally following the 16/8 method, then eating just one meal a day for a couple of days will increase your fasting time for those days. Another option is to move your mealtimes, having your last meal at 7pm, water-fasting the next day, and then eating at 7am on the third day.

Whichever way you decide to go, adding fasting days can do wonders for many bowel diseases.

It has been found that in people with IBS and IBD and other inflammatory gut conditions that the MMC does not function well. Patients with SIBO and IBS tend to have a third as many MMC phase III events, and the ones that they do have do not last as long. Adding total fast days to weekly, or fortnightly routines could go a long way to helping this situation and healing from these diseases.

Eradication of bacterial overgrowth has been shown to partially restore MMC function.

There may also be other reasons that the MMC is not working strongly. These can include the presence of autoimmune diseases, nerve damage, stress and narcotics including analgesic pain medications.

Stimulating the MMC

There are a group of products known as prokinetics. These are agents that improve gastrointestinal motility by increasing the frequency or the strength of contractions.

There are many drugs that fly under the banner of prokinetics, but many of them are only good for colonic movement (defecation). But drugs that focus on cholinergics, serotonin receptor agonists or motilin administration can induce phase 3 of the MMC. This could be useful in some serious settings.

Bitters are often used as prokinetics to stimulate the MMC more naturally. These are usually found as herbal tinctures and other preparations. One commercial preparation called *Iberogast* claims to be just this. Even a bitter drink such as coffee can do the job. Some products claim to increase bile flow and the manufacture of bile in the liver. Some of the strongest herbs for this are:

- Globe artichoke
- Greater celandine
- Gentian
- Dandelion Root
- Oregon Grape Root
- Wormwood

Take care with these herbs. It may be best to see a herbalist or other specialist about them before going ahead. In cases of gallstones, these herbs may be best avoided, or used very sparingly.

Only use prokinetics in small amounts. The taste on your tongue is all that is needed.

Traditionally, many cultures used bitters before meals, to get the digestive juices going. This is fine to do, but for our purposes here, the best time to take them would be around the time that MMC function is due to start, to help stimulate the process.

During your feeding times, eating foods high in vitamins K1 and K2 could also have a great impact on your gut health. It has been observed that those with IBD tend to have lower levels of vitamin K. Vitamin K has several positive effects on the gut as explained in the previous chapter on gut health.

Digestion

I mentioned earlier that digestion and the MMC motility are two sides of the same coin, because one makes a mess and the other cleans it up.

The other connection between these two functions is that they use the same neural network to function. Now that we have discussed the sweeping and cleaning action of the MMC, the next chapter will dive a little into digestion. Because there are so many aspects about digestion that are generally poorly understood, it may be worth spending some time to explain.

Many people who undergo surgeries for reflux disease often do so without identifying the real cause of the disease, leading not only to surgery, but a failure of the surgery soon after. In fact, the digestive failures mentioned in the next chapter could be the cause of most surgical failures. If you have ever been thinking to receive surgery for your acid reflux, then this next chapter may be worth your attention.

What you can do

Supporting the MMC

- Eat foods that are high in vitamin K1 and K2 (or supplement). Inform your doctor about this change in your nutrition.

- Incorporate fasting into your daily routine.

- Eat more nutrient-dense foods, so that you can eat less often.

- Try taking a small amount of bitters to promote the MMC cycle.

CHAPTER 8

GASTROPARESIS

One thing that is very frustrating for acid reflux patients, is cycling through all the treatments, only to find that there is no improvement in the condition. The usual treatments normally consist of testing for unbalanced microbes and testing of acid levels in the upper gastrointestinal region, and an endoscopy to observe any physical issues.

Normally the tests end there, but there is another group of tests that should be explored more often. These test the nerves of the upper GI system and the functionality of the stomach and the intestines. These could determine whether a condition known as gastroparesis exists.

Gastroparesis can cause acid reflux, and normally comes with a swathe of symptoms, but when patients don't present with these symptoms, many doctors automatically assume that gastroparesis is not a factor in the equation.

Unfortunately, not everyone experiences symptoms when gastroparesis is present, and for some people the only observable symptom is acid reflux.

The definition for gastroparesis states that it is a condition that affects the stomach muscles and prevents proper stomach emptying. But as we will see in a moment, the cause of gastroparesis is not so simple, and there are a number of tests that may need to be carried out to have a proper diagnosis.

The Digestive Process

Digestion is the most important function of the digestive system. Churning and mixing of food is an action that is performed in the stomach first, and then in the intestines.

Strong muscular digestive action begins in the stomach. It pushes the food back and forth under great pressure. This helps to tear the food apart to a small extent, but it also ensures that enzymes are working as effectively as they can possibly be. With this method they manage to get into every surface and crevice, outside and inside the food.

When the food begins to be released into the intestines, a new set of enzymes and bile are released to break the food down even more. The churning action of the intestines ensures that the enzymes here are also mixed in and are working effectively.

This digestive action of the stomach and the intestines should happen every time you eat.

Active Parts of the System

There are quite a number of parts that need to work together to make the stomach completely functional.

First, of course, there is the stomach. There are three sections to the stomach. The top dome-shaped section of the stomach is called the fundus. The main part of the stomach is the body and the lead up to the exit is called the antrum. The stomach is the star of the show, but its performance is determined by an intricate set of nerves that lead it around.

At the top and the bottom of the stomach are valves that stop food and acid from escaping the stomach. The entry into the top of the stomach is a valve called the lower esophageal sphincter (LES). Many people are convinced that a weak LES is the cause of reflux, but a weak LES is probably rarer than people tend to believe. In a moment we will discuss a common fault that causes the LES to fail.

The valve at the exit is called the pyloric sphincter, or pylorus. Pylorus means "Gateway" in Greek, and the pyloric sphincter is the gateway into the intestines. This exit is a small opening, measuring about 2cm. This valve is surrounded by thick loops of muscle and these hold tightly shut while food is being churned in the stomach. It opens only during the short moments when food is being pushed into the intestines by the stomach.

Many nerves are involved in regulating digestion in the stomach, including the main one, the vagus nerve, so-called because it 'wanders' around the internal organs, connecting to each one. The Latin word 'vagus' means 'wanderer'. And there are a number of other nerve-related parts, including some special cells called Interstitial Cells of Cajal (ICC).

These parts all work together to create a synchronized dance of sorts. There is a special timing to the dance, and if someone puts a foot wrong, the entire thing collapses.

It is easy to think that the stomach just sits there while it secretes acid to break down the food that is inside. After all, we don't feel a thing when it is working properly.

Instead, the stomach is extremely active, and cycles through a pattern of movements that churn the food to help mix and break it down.

A pacemaker that is located at the upper end of the stomach sends out electrical pulses to a network of nerves that surround the muscles of the stomach.

The nerves activate some special cells called the Interstitial Cells of Cajal (ICC). These accept the signals from the nerves, and then translate them into pulsing electrical frequencies to the muscles of the stomach. The ICCs remain in between the nerves and the muscles and are often described as the pacemaker cells of the gastrointestinal system, because they regulate the coordination within the complex system of muscles.

The ICCs lead the stomach through a churning cycle, which is a particular set of movements that it performs three times a minute.

First, it generates a circular movement around the main area of the stomach, and then it sends a wave down toward the lower end of the stomach. If it is time for food to move through to the intestines, then the pylorus will also get involved.

The pylorus normally remains shut, until the moment when the stomach sends a wave of motion toward the lower end of the stomach. At that exact moment, the pylorus will open large enough to let a small amount of the digested food into the intestines. It is a well-timed dance that needs to be executed with a certain amount of precision.

The speed of cycles and waves of the stomach action is important. It must be roughly three cycles per minute. Just one or two cycles is too slow, and 4 or more cycles is too fast.

Pressure inside the stomach

A badly-timed maneuver can result in enormous pressure inside the stomach.

The timing is important because it must match up with the opening of the pylorus which will also take place three times a minute. If the pylorus is closed when the stomach is pressing down on it, the pressure inside the stomach becomes so intense, that something has to give way.

The muscles of the LES (top of the stomach) can contract at a pressure of around 40mmHG. If everything inside the stomach is working properly, then the pressure inside the stomach should stay at less than 40mmHg. However, if the pressure inside the stomach builds up to around 44mmHg or more, then the LES will not be able to contain it. The pressure created inside the stomach is simply too high for the normal strength of the LES muscles, and the stomach contents are forced upward at high pressure, resulting in symptoms of acid reflux.

This fault in the timing is known as gastroparesis. There are several forms of gastroparesis, and most of them are caused by a faulty nerve system.

Gastroparesis of the stomach

One of the signs of gastroparesis is food sitting inside the stomach for too long. This is not because the stomach is inactive, but because the pylorus is closed the moment the stomach tries to push food into the intestine. The stomach may be trying to cycle 2 or 4 times per minute instead of 3.

Mistiming of the stomach/pylorus movements can delay the emptying of the stomach by hours. In a normal case, 50% of the stomach contents will be gone after 2 hours, and after 4 hours only 10% is still left.

In the case of gastroparesis, most of the food may still be in the stomach after the initial 2 hours have passed. This delay in gastric emptying can be quite benign for some people, and can be present without any symptoms at all, but for others the reaction to consumption of food is severe.

Gastroparesis of the pylorus

Another way that gastroparesis can occur is if the pylorus is at fault. Perhaps the stomach is functioning perfectly fine, but the pylorus is not accepting the stomach contents into the intestines.

This could be because the pylorus opening is out of sync, or because there is a blockage, such as a tumor, scar tissue, or an ulcer that has caused some swelling.

Gastroparesis of the intestines

A third type of gastroparesis can affect the muscular action of the intestines.

In many people, the nerve system has been damaged, and the intestines fail to move. This can affect both movements of the intestines – the action to churn food, and the action to move food along, down the line.

Overarching Symptoms of Gastroparesis

There are many symptoms and conditions that are associated with gastroparesis.

Gastroparesis caused by the stomach or the pylorus can result in nausea, vomiting, bloating, indigestion and acid reflux. It is common to feel full after eating very little, or to have a complete loss of appetite altogether. For many people, the lack of food, and the inability to eat, can lead to malnutrition, while the indigestible elements, such as fiber can form stone-like objects in the stomach, called bezoars, which can be life-threatening.

In the intestines, a lack of action can give a feeling of being backed up or result in abdominal pain. Intestinal movement that is too slow or sluggish, usually results in constipation. And in addition to this, bacterial overgrowth or SIBO can also take hold. It particularly becomes an issue that is difficult to treat when gastroparesis is one of the causes. If gastroparesis of the intestines has set in, the MMC may not be functioning properly.

For many people gastroparesis presents no symptoms at all. Acid reflux may be the only sign. And how many doctors test for gastroparesis as the cause of acid reflux? Gastroparesis is often not tested in people who have acid reflux. Many people do not experience the symptoms of gastroparesis, but the evidence of it may still be found if proper testing is done. And it should be done if all other avenues of acid reflux treatment have failed.

Why testing is important

It is crucial to test for gastroparesis for two reasons. One is to identify or eliminate gastroparesis as a condition causing your acid reflux. If it is caused by gastroparesis, you may be able to receive the proper treatment for gastroparesis, and hopefully solve your problem.

The second reason is that an undiagnosed condition can lead to treatment disasters. There have been reported cases where patients have undergone surgery to eliminate reflux, only to find that the surgery fails, because the real cause of reflux was gastroparesis.

Why would surgery fail? Current reflux surgeries aim to add support to the LES muscle if it is abnormally weak. If the real cause of the reflux is from gastroparesis, then the pressure in the stomach can still become high enough to squeeze past the LES. Stomach pressure from gastroparesis will overcome the strength of any surgical procedure.

An exceptionally large number of fundoplication surgeries (and other reflux surgeries) end up as failures. Is this just bad luck? It is more likely to be a faulty diagnosis, or a common failure to test for gastroparesis. A surgical procedure for reflux should not be performed when gastroparesis is the true cause.

How to Test for Gastroparesis

1. Test pressure of the LES. Unfortunately, the corresponding pressure inside the stomach cannot be tested, so other tests are needed here to determine why stomach contents are getting past the LES.

2. Test electrical pulses of the stomach with an electrogastrogram. This can show that the stomach and the pylorus are both moving at the same rate and are generating impulses at the proper rate of three cycles per minute.

3. Have a gastric emptying test to determine that food is moving out of the stomach at the correct rate. If the timing of the stomach and pylorus are correct, the stomach should be emptying. If it is not emptying properly, despite good timing, there may be some type of blockage obstructing the movement of food.

4. Endoscopy. An endoscopy is necessary to find out what types of obstructions may exist. In some cases, there is no visible structural damage to the pylorus, but the muscles are too tight to allow it to open fully.

5. Report your medications. There are a number of medications that slow the rate of stomach emptying. This could lead to false positives in the tests if your doctor is unaware. Some common medications that can affect gastric emptying are these:
   a. Opioid pain relievers
   b. Some antidepressants
   c. High Blood Pressure Medications
   d. Allergy Medications

Causes of Gastroparesis

"Paresis" comes from a Greek word, meaning 'partial paralysis'. This tends to indicate that the main causes of gastroparesis are due to loss of nerve function. The nervous system is a common thread that controls both types of intestinal function: the digestive functions and the migrating motor complex.

There are numerous ways that the nervous system can be damaged. Sadly, one cause of nerve damage, especially the vagus nerve, can occur during medical procedures, such as endoscopies. There are always dangers with any medical procedure, and although this type of error is uncommon, it is good to be aware of this possibility. Find a doctor that you feel confident with.

Inflammation is a common cause of just about any dysfunction in the body, and gastroparesis can be one of them.

Diabetes is always associated with nerve damage. Nerve damage in the hands and feet is well-known, but many people don't realize that diabetes can also affect the nerves in the gastro-intestinal tract, and the ICC cells in the stomach. In fact, insulin resistance in any form, whether you have diabetes or not, has the potential to lead to nerve damage in the digestive system.

One test that is rarely conducted on patients, is measurement of the level of insulin circulating in the blood. Most doctors will normally test for blood-sugar, and then make assumptions about insulin levels, but people who have normal blood-sugar levels can still have excessive insulin levels. Studies have found that high insulin levels can slow the intestinal system by up to forty percent!

Hopefully, you are underway with a low-carb diet as outlined in previous chapters. This is one of the best ways to eventually normalize blood sugar, insulin and other hormones.

In books two and three of this *Acid Reflux Formula* series, we will also be discussing the role that foods and the immune system can play in damage to the body. Various neurological diseases such as Parkinson's or Multiple Sclerosis can have a direct impact on the immune system, as can any type of autoimmune disease. There are many people that are completely unaware that they are on the way to developing autoimmune diseases, and every year the number of people with autoimmune diseases is growing.

One particular condition, an underactive thyroid, whether caused by autoimmune disease or not, will cause the digestive system to become sluggish, and could also lead to a diagnosis of gastroparesis.

Solutions for Gastroparesis

Most of these diseases can be overcome, if conditions are not too advanced, and some of the damage could possibly be reversed. This will differ from person to person, of course!

The good news is that if nerves are only slightly damaged, there is the possibility that they can grow back. This is the case for a stomach that has lost its timing, as well as an intestinal section that is not moving properly.

In the cases of pyloric obstructions, a surgical procedure may need to be performed to allow the pylorus to open again. Different types of procedures are available including a temporary one, where Botox is used to paralyze the pyloric muscles, keeping them open until the Botox wears off (approximately three months).

Other risky procedures on the pylorus involve cutting the muscles to prevent them from closing completely, but a novel approach is a procedure where a balloon is used to stretch the muscles of the pylorus. This has the effect of widening the aperture of the pyloric opening, and apparently comes without any significant side effects.

Gastroparesis can be life-changing, but in many cases, with good guidance it is something that can be overcome. Hopefully, you have been able to maintain your low-carb diet to support your metabolic system and your nervous system because this will have a great impact on the strength of the condition and whether it can be resolved.

Dealing with intestinal and functional issues is important because in the next chapter we will be discussing a factor that relies on good intestinal functionality. If your intestinal system is fully functional, but you are still experiencing acid reflux, then the next chapter will be talking about the trigger that helps the LES to close tightly and increase the digestive capacity of the entire gastrointestinal system.

What You Can Do

Supporting gastroparesis

- Follow a low carb diet
  - Damage from insulin resistance can sometimes be reversed with a persistent low-carb diet that can allow some nerve regrowth in some people.

- Take steps to support Your Nervous system
  - Take steps to activate the vagus nerve regularly. This includes relaxation, meditation, casual walking, singing, laughing, playing with pets, as well as many other activities.

Testing for gastroparesis

- HOMA-IR test for insulin resistance and for abnormal insulin levels.
- Electrogastrogram to test the action and timing of the stomach.
- Gastric Emptying Test to confirm that stomach contents are emptying in a timely manner.
- Endoscopy. If the cause of gastroparesis is still unknown, an endoscopy may be needed to observe any physical obstructions and other irregularities in the stomach.

CHAPTER 9

RAISE YOUR ACID LEVELS

2000 years ago, Hippocrates said that all disease begins in the gut. In other words, the gut is the stronghold of the body. Modern doctors are amazed at his insight into health, but what Hippocrates did not know is that the strength of the gut comes from hydrochloric acid (HCl). HCl is the powerhouse of the entire digestive system. Without it nothing can function.

You may have heard that humans can survive without stomach acid, and it is true that we can survive. But we survive with a poor quality of life. Life without stomach acid leads to a slow and painful demise, filled with diseases and an unshakable feeling of depression.

Our bodies are designed to have acid for a reason. One reason is that it acts as a trigger for other hormones in our bodies, and the other reason is that we cannot absorb all our nutrients without it. Have you ever tried taking vitamin supplements, hoping that it will counteract a lack of stomach acid? Did you know that many vitamins and minerals cannot be absorbed without acid?

Acid breaks down proteins, and other food structures that encase the vitamins that we need. And then it helps the body to absorb those nutrients. It also helps to keep our bodies safe from undigested food, which can eventually lead to serious chronic diseases like autoimmune disease.

Have you ever developed weak fingernails, or noticed your vision degenerating earlier than it should? Or have you suffered from asthma as a child? Lack of stomach acid can be the leading cause of many strange and random symptoms that probably seem minor at first glance.

Depression and anxiety are quite common complaints, and I often hear questions about the relationship between acid reflux and depression. There are many reasons for this relationship, but the major one is because of low stomach acid.

If you are not producing enough stomach acid, there could be many reasons why this is happening. It could be a physical problem where the acid-producing cells of the stomach have died. It could be caused by a fault or by degeneration of the nervous system, or a lack of the right micronutrients. It can even be dependent on your mood.

The two most common causes of poor acid secretion (other than gastritis) are a lack of protein absorption and having an unrelaxed emotional state.

Fortunately, most of these diseases of low stomach acid can be reversed over time, with proper treatment, which must include restoring the proper pH level in the stomach.

How Digestion Begins

In order to understand how to raise stomach acid levels, it is good to understand how the digestive system works. A lot of your actions, routines and relationships are involved in producing stomach acid, so a short explanation of the digestive process could help you to make changes to your lifestyle.

It all begins with the nervous system. Eating food is not something that should be dissociated from your surroundings. The body is designed to digest food when it is relaxed, and when the mind is in a state of calm and safety.

Eating with friends and family are the best surroundings to have, where laughing and joking indicate a sense of creativity. In these situations, the vagus nerve that travels from the brain to all the organs in the gut, including the stomach, is being activated. This is the perfect time for a meal.

This is where we enter the first phase of digestion: The cephalic phase. This is where all the senses become involved in the meal before you even start to eat. Mealtimes normally conjure up thoughts of the upcoming meal. If you are really hungry, the anticipation at this point can be powerful, and as the smells waft past, and the sight of the food looks appealing, something changes in your brain.

A signal is sent through the vagus nerve to prepare the stomach for food. The stomach starts producing HCl in a large quantity, before you have even had your first bite. This phase of digestion, including the taste and texture of the meal, can account for up to 20% of the production of HCl in the stomach.

Once you have swallowed your first bite, the second phase of digestion can begin. This is the gastric phase and is dependent on the feedback about the food from receptors in the stomach.

HCl and acidity level

Every time you swallow more of your meal, the food dilutes the HCl in the stomach, so that the whole environment becomes less acidic. But the pH must remain exceptionally low, between 1 and 2. So, the stomach uses a feedback system to control the pH of its contents. Receptors in the gut monitor the acid levels and send out signals accordingly. If the pH rises too high (low acid), the stomach sends out the hormone, Gastrin, into the bloodstream.

Gastrin does two things. Firstly, it promotes the production of HCL from the parietal cells (acid-producing cells) of the stomach. This adds more acid to the food. And secondly, it promotes contractions of smooth muscles in the stomach for better digestion. The muscles of the stomach compress and grind the food to help break it down.

This is where things get slightly complicated, but it may be worth knowing about it. There are 2 ways for HCl production to be stimulated from the parietal cells. The first is by the hormone Gastrin, and the second is by histamine molecules.

By itself, gastrin only has an extremely limited effect on the parietal cells. In its presence, the cells will produce only a small amount of HCl. But gastrin also stimulates the production of histamine (from ECL cells), and it is histamine that has the greatest impact on HCl production from the parietal cells. Histamine is the primary driver of acid production.

You may have heard about, or even relied on H2 blocker medications to help suppress the acid levels in your stomach. The way they work is by blocking the histamine receptors on the parietal cells, so that the presence of histamine goes undetected. Without the effect of histamine, the bulk of the acid production disappears. With these medications, there is still a small amount of acid being produced, because gastrin is still there, stimulating the parietal cells to work.

When it comes to PPI drugs the effect is much greater. PPI drugs target the parietal cells and block their ability to produce HCl altogether. The presence of gastrin and histamine cannot wake them up, and so the result can be production of little to no acid at all. When there is not enough acid being produced, the pH rises, and the strength of the acid is weak. The medications do not stop the stomach from trying to change the situation. The stomach continues its efforts to produce more HCl, so that the contents of the stomach can be digested. The stomach is registering a high pH – it needs to be low – so it continues to send out gastrin with the goal of lowering the pH to where it should be. If the parietal cells are unable to produce acid, then the gastrin levels continue to rise.

This creates a situation called *hypergastrinemia* where too much gastrin can lead to ulcers and to stomach cancer. It also causes the rebound effect that we mentioned in chapter 4.

In a normal functional stomach, gastrin would stimulate the production of HCl, lower the acidity, and then the stomach would stop producing more gastrin.

HCl signals production of digestive products

Acid is not the only substance that breaks down food in the stomach. There are a number of other products that need to be manufactured if we are going to be able to digest our food properly. When acid levels are high, some of the other cells in the stomach are stimulated to produce other substances, to help improve digestive capacity.

147

The first is pepsin. It begins life as a small molecule called pepsinogen, but when it encounters acid, it changes to its destructive, meat-eating form, pepsin. HCl cannot completely digest many foods on its own, and pepsin has the power to reduce protein foods into liquids in a short space of time.

Pepsin is dependent on HCl to give it the power to do its digestive work. As the pH rises to 3, 4 or 5, pepsinogen becomes weaker and weaker, and proteins take much longer to digest properly. The optimal pH for pepsin to work is 1.8. At this level, pepsin can reduce a meaty meal into liquid in about an hour.

Another molecule that depends on high acidity is intrinsic factor. This molecule is only formed when stomach pH is low, where it should be, and it is created to perform just one specific task in the digestive system. Intrinsic factor is inactive in the stomach, but comes to life in the alkaline environment of the intestines. In this environment it clings to the B12 molecules and carries them all the way to the final section of the small intestines, the ileum, where both particles are absorbed into the epithelial cells. From here, B12 is supplied to the rest of the body. Without proper HCl levels, intrinsic factor would never be produced, and the body can be starved of this essential vitamin.

In addition to this, proper HCl levels trigger the release of a thicker mucus layer to protect the lining of the stomach.

HCl and bioavailability

There are many minerals and vitamins that could not possibly be absorbed into the body's bloodstream if HCl was not there to make them available. This is exactly why preventing acid in the stomach leads to malnutrition. This process is easy to see in the case of iron, calcium and vitamin B12.

Before iron can be absorbed, it needs to be released from its food matrix. This is especially the case with plants, where iron is bound up tightly with other molecules. Once the task of releasing the iron has taken place, it then needs to be absorbed. The form of iron in food makes a big difference. Animal products contain a form called heme-iron, and this can be absorbed easily, even if the acid levels are poor. The iron from plants, called non-heme iron, is not so easy to digest. If acid levels drop too low at any time, then the iron floats around as unabsorbable ferrous salts, but in a highly acidic solution it is possible for the body to use it. This example shows why acid needs to be strong from beginning to end of the breakdown process in the stomach. Antacids at any point will render this type of iron as lost.

The same goes for calcium. This mineral needs to be cleaved from the other substances that are binding it in the food. In the 1960s it was discovered that people who were on calcium supplements continued to be deficient in calcium if their stomach acid was low. As with iron, HCl need to be strong enough to extract calcium from the matrix that is binding it, and then continue to be strong enough to keep the calcium in an absorbable form.

B12 is found in animal products and is usually found bound up with protein molecules. A number of steps need to occur before we can absorb B12, and all of them rely on having a strong level of HCl in the stomach.

In order to extract the B12, stomach acid needs to be strong enough to activate pepsin to a significant degree. Together, acid and pepsin break down the protein structure so that B12 can be released into the acid solution. HCl also needs to be strong enough to stimulate the production of intrinsic factor from the cells of the stomach, because once these particles move into the intestines, B12 and intrinsic factor bind together so that B12 can be absorbed at the end of the small intestine. If any step of this process does not occur, then B12 does not get absorbed.

These same principles apply to most of the vitamins and minerals, including zinc, A, E and B vitamins. At the least, anything that is bound to proteins or other substances will need to be extracted before it can easily be absorbed.

HCl stimulates bile and pancreatic enzymes

Now we are moving out of the stomach and into the intestines. The effect of HCl is not confined to the stomach. It is essential for the proper functionality of the digestive processes further down the line.

After the stomach, food makes its way into the first part of the small intestines, the Duodenum. Receptors in the duodenum detect the presence of HCl, which triggers the digestive events of the small intestines.

Firstly, the duodenum produces GIP (Gastric Inhibitory Peptide), which slows down the emptying of the stomach into the intestines. We want the stomach contents to start emptying out in a controlled manner, and not in a flood of food and acid.

The duodenum contains receptors that detect the presence of amino acids (proteins) and fats in the food. If these particles are present, the duodenum produces a hormone called Cholecystokinin (CCK). CCK stimulates the gallbladder to contract, releasing bile into the intestines. Bile neutralizes the acid and emulsifies fats so that they can be digested by pancreatic enzymes.

CCK also stimulates the pancreas to release digestive enzymes. These break down the food particles even further, so that they can be absorbed into the bloodstream.

The duodenum also detects the pH of the food. When it detects acid, it sends out another hormone called secretin. Secretin acts on the pancreas to secrete bicarbonate, and alkaline substance which assists in neutralizing the pH of the food that has just arrived from the stomach.

Without high levels of HCl in the food, these steps would not happen, and the organs would not respond strongly to food that is entering the system. Without acid, the food in the stomach remains undigested, and the enzymes from the intestines don't get released in the volumes that are needed. It is hardly surprising that malnutrition can be an issue when acid levels are not adequate.

Barrier to pathogens

HCl also has another important role that is not completely understood. It keeps intestinal populations of microbes under control.

The intestines house populations of microbes that are supposed to live in particular areas. The small intestines normally house very few microbes, and the large intestine is home to all the bacteria that are supposed to be beneficial to our health.

When HCl is too low, populations of bacteria can become overgrown in the small intestine, and some microbes begin to live in areas that they normally would not. Also, the bacteria from the colon begin to migrate into the small intestine. This migration and overgrowth is known as SIBO and is the cause of a lot of intestinal discomfort.

When HCl in the stomach is at optimal levels, the populations in the intestines go back to normal. This may be to do with greater secretion of pancreatic enzymes and bile, but science has not yet found the true answers to this phenomenon.

The other major function of HCl is to provide what some people call the 'acid barrier'. Most microbes cannot live in an environment as acidic as our stomachs, so with normal levels of HCl, human stomachs are almost entirely sterile. No microbes can live there (with the exception of H.Pylori).

This also means that microbes should not be able to travel up into the mouth from the intestines, nor down into the intestines from the mouth.

This is important because we are surrounded by thousands of different types of bacteria outside our bodies. These can all be harmless if they are living in the areas that they are meant to be. For example, the bacteria that live on our skin are harmless while they are on the skin, but if they enter the intestines or our bloodstream, the results can be fatal. There are hundreds of bacteria that live in our mouths and throats, but if they remain there and don't pass through the stomach into the intestines, then we can avoid many illnesses.

On the other hand, it is important that microbes from the inside do not make their way up through the stomach. There are theories about asthma being the cause of pathogens that have been allowed to travel up from the intestines, because the pH of the stomach was not strong enough to hold them back.

There is also another problem. When stomach acid is too low, microbes can move into the stomach and interfere with the digestive process. They can then steal vitamins and minerals from us, to use for themselves. This is yet another one of the ways that a lack of stomach acid can lead to nutrient deficiencies.

Determining Your HCl Levels

Stomach acid production tends to decline as we age. The acid-producing cells of the stomach seem to die off over time, leading to smaller and smaller acid amounts. But it is not all about old age. Low stomach acid has been observed in people of all ages, including children.

It is a good idea to determine the reason why you might not be producing enough HCl.

Remember that diagnosing a lack of acid in your stomach should be the first step in correcting the deficiency. This will show whether your stomach can produce HCl, and whether it is healthy enough to take acid supplements.

A lack of stomach acid can be caused by a number of conditions. These can include the development of gastritis, or atrophic gastritis, or any number of diseases that can have an effect of the function of the stomach, including thyroid problems, autoimmune diseases, nerve troubles or even trauma or emotional troubles.

For a list of tests that can be done at home and with the aid of a physician, see the appendix to chapter nine.

Once a diagnosis has been reached, a test that determines the likely levels of vitamins and minerals in your system may be a next step. This can include a stool test to determine whether vitamins, minerals and proteins/fats are being digested properly in your system, or if they are simply being passed out each time that you eat.

Ways to Increase Acid in the Stomach

There are 4 ways to increase acidity in the stomach. Not all of them are equal, though. Let us examine them:

First Method – supplementing HCl and pepsin

- Consume capsules that contain HCl and pepsin

If you want to have your digestion upregulated as soon as possible, the best method, of course, is to take HCl capsules. If your stomach is not producing enough HCl, for any reason at all, then you will need to have adequate levels to trigger the cascade of digestive events that you need.

Taking HCl capsules is a natural and safe way to increase your digestive capacity. It is not a drug that changes the way that your body works, so there are no real side-effects. It is simply there to replace what is missing in your stomach.

This is the preferred method to fix digestive capacity. Because it is instantaneous, and you can begin absorbing the right nutrients straight away, building up the vitamins and minerals that you have been missing out on up to this point. Better nutrition can help improve your gut's ability to digest food and can also help your nervous system to eventually improve your relaxation.

The other methods in this section take some time to begin working. I would not forego taking HCl supplement in favor of the other methods. Instead, you can combine them with your HCl supplementation for greater benefit.

Second Method – approach to food

- Rest and digest
- Cephalic Phase of digestion
  - Relax and take time
  - Having the meal with friends
  - Laugh, joke and have fun
  - Thoughts of food
  - Smell of the food
  - Flavor of the food

Some may laugh that this approach to digestion, but the plain fact is that the body and mind are wired to work this way. If you are the type of person that eats meals on the go, or gulps food down as quickly as possible, in serious environments, you will never, ever achieve 100% digestive capacity.

Personally, I also watch the stress count on my smart watch to gauge my level of relaxation. I observe how much my stress levels change in different environments and activities, and how they change with different foods. The more relaxed you are, the more quickly a lack of digestive capacity can turn around. If you are normally not completely relaxed in your eating environment, then breaking this habit may take some time to correct.

Third Method – vitamin and mineral supplements

- Vitamins and minerals that are low in the body
- L-Lysine
- B-complex, especially B12

Reflux often occurs because our bodies have not received the nutrition that we need to maintain proper digestive function. If you can identify vitamins and minerals in deficit, through tests that are available, then you may be able to target these.

Replenishing vitamins and minerals takes time to work. The effects will not be immediate. In addition to this, taking supplements orally can work particularly slowly, especially if your digestion is not good, because the body can only take in a certain amount at a time. Intravenous sources of vitamins are faster and more effective.

Aside from general vitamin deficiencies, some supplements that tend to help with digestive capacity are L-lysine, vitamin B12 and some of the B-complex vitamins.

Fourth Method – natural medicinal remedies

- diluted lemon or vinegar prior to meals
- the use of herbal bitters
  - Centaurium minus or erythraea (common or red centaury)
  - Gentiana lutea, (gentian)

- Zingiber officinale (ginger)
- Piper nigrum (black pepper)
- Capsicum annum (cayenne)

These natural remedies, along with some others, are thought to raise HCl production.

Natural remedies of this type do not work for everyone, and in many cases may even make reflux worse. This was the case for me, and I talk about this more in the section about nutrition. The best course of action to take would be to avoid these natural remedies until your digestion has improved and stabilized. You would then have the option to experiment with them to see if they can maintain your digestive capacity as an alternative to HCL supplementation, if this were something that you would like to try out.

Choosing an HCl Supplement

There are a lot of different brands of HCl on the market, but they are not all the same. The active ingredient might always be HCl, but the fillers and binders and extra ingredients are what can make the difference.

1. Choose a product that is HCl + Pepsin. Some people may do well by choosing a supplement that does not include pepsin, but most people will benefit from the extra pepsin included in the supplement.

2. Avoid supplements that contain unnecessary fillers and binders, especially if they are made from milk, such as lactose or casein. Many people develop reflux from these ingredients, and having them included in a supplement, like this one, could make your reflux worse, not better.

3. Avoid supplements with other plant-based enzymes such as bromelain and papain. It is best to steer clear of these types of substances until digestion improves. They are unnecessary and not particularly effective, and it is best not to invite trouble with ingredients that could possibly cause a reaction of any type. At this stage, we only want HCl and pepsin.

It is good to be aware that there are two types of HCl on the market. One is called betaine hydrochloride, and the other is glutamic acid hydrochloride. The betaine and the glutamic acid components are simply carriers for the HCL, so that it can be easily packaged into a capsule. Betaine is a much smaller molecule, so a lot more HCl can fit into a capsule when it is accompanied by betaine rather than glutamic acid.

The most common of these two supplements is betaine HCl. If you find that you are not reacting well to the supplement you are taking, check for the purity of the product. Write to the company, if you must, to check if there are any hidden fillers that you don't know about.

If you are still having problems with your chosen supplement, you can try another brand, or you can change the version of the acid. If you are using a betaine version, then switch to a glutamic acid version, and vice versa. Some people react to one type of HCL but are fine with the other.

Determining the Dosage

How much HCl will you need to digest a meal properly? Are you extremely deficient, or only slightly deficient?

Some factors will change the amount you take, such as the type of food you are eating and how much you are eating at a meal.

Assuming that you are having meals of roughly the same size each time you eat, here is one method that you can use. When you use HCl, you need to look out for a feeling of warmth in the stomach. When you feel this, you can step down the number of capsules that you take.

1. Take 1 capsule part-way through your meal. If everything goes well, and you don't feel any 'warmth' in the stomach, then take 2 capsules part-way through your meals on the next day. Look for the same signs. If you find nothing, then take 3 with meals on the next day.

2. If you are taking multiple capsules at a meal, then space them out through the meal. Don't take them all at once.

3. If you find that you are experiencing that "warm" feeling during a meal, then stop taking capsules, and at the next meal, take the same number of capsules, minus one. For example, if you reach 6 capsules and experience some warmth, then you would take only 5 capsules at the following meal.

4. It is best to take no more than 7 capsules that contain 650mg of HCl per capsule. This would be 4550mg at one single meal. In any case, a normal stomach should be able to produce more than this amount.

Caution About Using HCl

Using HCl is safe to use because it is exactly what the body uses, and in this sense it is natural. However, you need to know when to avoid it. The stomach normally keeps a thick coating of mucus to protect the stomach walls from being damaged by the acid. If this mucus lining has been compromised, then you should seek some help before trying HCl supplements.

These circumstances can include when an ulcer exists or there is other damage to the stomach lining. There are other occasions where food or supplements can thin out the mucus lining, increasing the chances of damage to the stomach.

- Never take HCl if you are taking painkillers of any type, including NSAIDs, Aspirin, Ibuprofen, Tylenol, etc. These products thin the mucus layer on the stomach, leaving it open to damage.

- If you are taking any other medications that could be affecting the gut lining, or the mucus on the gut lining, then talk to a physician about your options.

- If you are diagnosed with gastritis, or atrophic gastritis, then you may not be able to produce the amount of mucus required to protect the lining of the stomach. HCl can cause some discomfort in this case, and you should work through this condition with a doctor.

- Good nutrition can have a big impact on the effectiveness of HCl. Avoiding foods that are difficult to digest is an effective move, as well as foods that may thin the lining of the stomach. You can find a lot more information about this in book two of this series.

What You Can Do

- Eat meals with friends and family in a relaxed environment.

- Consider taking HCl supplements to improve digestion.

- Improve the vitamin and mineral balance in your body.

Tests for Low Stomach acid

- See the appendix for chapter nine for a list of tests to determine whether your HCl levels are healthy.

Further Reading

- *Why Stomach Acid is Good for You* by Dr Jonathan Wright

CONCLUSION

If you have never previously investigated improving your health by taking the steps outlined in this book, then it can be a lot to take in. I guarantee that it becomes second nature over time.

There have been a lot of words and discussion points throughout the book. It is easy to lose sight of the goal when bombarded with a lot of ideas. It might be worth making a short summary of all the suggestions made so far.

First, we raised the topic of body-fat, and the type of body fat that affects reflux the most. This answered the question about whether the fat that you have in and around your body is or isn't contributing to your reflux.

There was no action to take in chapter one because chapter two was an extension on the causes of body fat and other metabolic disorders that can lead to reflux disease. Internal body fat may be one of the signs of a decline in metabolic health.

In chapter three we provided the answer to excess body fat and metabolic decline in three grades of diet that have been shown to improve metabolic function. These diets provide the foundation that support all other steps throughout this book.

Next, we discussed why eliminating acid-suppressing drugs is essential to overcoming reflux and provided a routine that can help you to ween off the medications.

In chapters four, five and six we began the process of fixing various aspects of the gut, by supporting the health of the gut lining, saving your gut microbiota and providing balance to it, and making the most of your gut-cleansing system. These steps can only succeed in conjunction with the diet from chapter three. They aim to minimize the gut-related diseases as well as overproduction of histamines and immune responses that can exacerbate gut health issues.

In an intervening chapter I suggested that it may be worth considering the possibility of gastroparesis as a cause of reflux disease, after which we launched into chapter nine to find ways to normalize the levels of acid in the stomach to upregulate the digestive capacity of the gut and to provide extra protection from microbial overgrowth.

Many people tend to focus on individual food triggers when trying to manage reflux disease, without attending to proper support of the body. The steps provided here cannot be separated from such a mission and must be maintained no matter which diet variations you may follow.

Moving into Dietary Support

Although supporting the function of the body's systems is the first priority, diet could not be excluded from this book. In a sense, the diet that was provided was done so to help support the way that the body functions – that is, the metabolic functions.

If the methods in this book have not cured your reflux already, then there may be some food sensitivities that you need to identify or overcome.

As we move into book two, the basic principles of the diet will not change from what we have established here, but the foods that you need to eat may change immensely.

For reflux patients, very few dietary guidelines are provided by the medical system to help manage the disease. There are a few specific foods that are normally avoided, and it is up to you to find your way through the maze of foods to find out whether they will be of benefit, or whether they will make your condition worse. Unfortunately, most people are not provided with the basics that we have discussed here already, and so determining whether a food is reflux-friendly or not becomes incredibly complicated.

Most people with reflux end up with a terrible nutritional status and a poor understanding of how different foods could be affecting their health. There are no right or wrong answers when it comes to nutrition, and it all comes down to what works best for you. There are some especially important details that are never revealed in nutritional circles, and these facts can make all the difference to the trajectory of your health.

Some of these facts are beginning to become more widely known, such as the toxicity of spinach or the dangers of gluten. Some of the foods that were previously touted as being the 'healthiest' are now being avoided by many people.

For example, green smoothies made with spinach can contribute to kidney stones and joint issues as well as the deterioration of other organs if it is consumed in excess or too regularly. Gluten can create problems with the skin, the gut, nutritional balances and auto-immune diseases. Most people know this about gluten, but don't realize that gluten-like proteins are also found in other products that include corn and oats.

We will discuss nutritional strategies that can build upon the low-carb diets that we have discussed here already, and we will be investigating the food groups that you will need to know about in order to understand your own symptoms. You will also find out why not all elimination diets work, what a true elimination diet really is, and why the results of some elimination diets don't apply in all situations.

The information here in book one has provided a foundation that should be maintained consistently while experimenting with the different food types and their effects on your body. I hope that the information in the next book provides as much value to your own quest to overcome reflux as it has for me.

GLOSSARY OF TERMS

Achlorhydria	A medical term describing a lack of any HCl production in the stomach.
BMI	Body Mass Index. A basic formula using height and weight to categorize a person's weight as underweight, normal weight or overweight. It is a very poor indicator of these classifications.
Cholecystokinin (CCK)	A hormone produced by the duodenum that stimulates the gallbladder to release bile and for the pancreas to release enzymes for digestion.
Duodenum	The very first section of the small intestines that is just outside the stomach.
Esophagus	Part of the digestive tract, it is a long muscular tube that transports food from the mouth to the stomach.
Gallbladder	Digestive organ that collects bile and distributes it as needed.
Gastrointestinal tract	This refers to the entire digestive path, from the mouth, to the esophagus, stomach and the intestines.
Glucagon	A hormone that signals the release of more glucose from the liver.

Glucose

A simple sugar, or carbohydrate, that the body uses for energy.

HCl

Hydrochloric Acid. This is the form of acid that the stomach uses to digest food.

Hypochlorhydria

A medical term that indicates low levels, or insufficient levels, of stomach acid.

Ileum

The third, or final, section of the small intestines that leads into the large intestine.

Insulin

A hormone that the body uses to feed glucose and other nutrients to cells. It is an anabolic hormone that promotes growth. Cells of the body can be sensitive or resistant to insulin.

Insulin Resistance

The inability for insulin to have its desired effect on cells of the body.

Intestines

Digestive organ, 5-10m in length. It carries out many functions including breakdown of food particles, absorption of nutrients, housing of beneficial bacteria and protection from pathogens.

Intrinsic Factor

This term was created by William B. Castle in the 1920s when his research into pernicious anemia indicated that two factors were involved: One created inside the body (intrinsic) and one outside the body (extrinsic). The extrinsic factor was later discovered to be B12 which is needed in the diet, and the intrinsic factor continued to be known as intrinsic factor.

Jejunum	The second, or middle, section of the small intestines.
Keotgenic Diet	A diet that promotes the production of ketones by the liver when carbohydrate consumption is very low.
Ketones	Particles produced from fat by the liver. Ketones are used by cells of the body to produce energy.
Ketosis	When the body begins to produce ketones for energy production, it can be said to be in a state of ketosis.
LES	Lower Esophageal Sphincter. This is a muscle at the top of the stomach that prevents food and acid from regurgitating back into the esophagus and the mouth.
MMC	Migrating Motor Complex. This is a function of the intestines to move contents and to clean the system.
NSAID	Non-steroidal Anti-Inflammatory Drug.
Pancreas	Digestive organ that secretes enzymes for the breakdown of proteins, carbohydrates and fats.
Parietal Cells	Cells of the stomach that produce the acid that we need for digestion.
pH	Power of Hydrogen. A scientific scale used to measure the acidity or alkalinity of a substance. It ranges from 0-14 but extremely strong substances can register outside the

extremes of the range. A low pH is more acid and a higher pH is more alkaline.

Secretin

A hormone produced by the duodenum that stimulates the pancreas to produce bicarbonate to neutralize the acidity of contents leaving the stomach.

Stomach

Digestive organ that breaks down food into a paste or liquid to prepare for further digestive processes in the digestive tract.

Subcutaneous Fat

Fat stored under the skin.

Vagus Nerve

A major nerve that extends from the brain and connects to all the digestive organs in the body. It is activated in times of rest.

Visceral Fat

Fat stored in the abdomen.

APPENDIX TO CHAPTER 1

Tests for Inflammation

Inflammation cannot be measured directly, but when it occurs, certain changes happen in the body. Doctors can test for the following tests to determine whether inflammation is creating issues. This list is for your interest and for your own research. There is almost no reason to have any of these tests done to test for inflammation unless there is a particular concern that needs investigation:

- Hs-CRP – C-Reactive Protein Test
  - This is probably the best test to show that inflammation is already present in your system.

- HbA1C – Long-term blood sugar levels
  - This simply gives an indication of the blood sugar levels over the last 3 months.
  - High result implies increased risk of inflammation and age-related chronic diseases

- Fasting Insulin
  - This is a good test when combined with blood sugar testing, and can indicate the state of your metabolic health.

- Serum Ferritin
  - Elevated serum Ferritin may indicate inflammation, liver disease, autoimmune disease and cancer.

- Red Blood Cell Width

- o The size of the blood cells is connected with maturation of the cells
- o High levels may be a sign that underlying inflammation has impacted the development of red blood cells

- Homocysteine Levels
  - o Elevated homocysteine levels may indicate inflammation and acute coronary syndrome.

- ESR – Erythrocyte Sedimentation Rate
  - o This test measures the rate at which your red blood cells in anti-coagulated whole blood go down in a standardized tube over the period of one hour.
  - o Also, a high number of platelets in the blood and the stickiness of the blood may indicate inflammation in the body.

- LDH – Lactate Dehydrogenase
  - o This is an enzyme that supports metabolic functions in the body. High levels may indicate inflammation is present.

- NLR – Neutrophil-Lymphocyte Ratio
  - o The ratio of Neutrophils to Lymphocytes will change over time when the body is dealing with chronic inflammation and stress. When Neutrophils are double the amount of lymphocytes, this is a sign of chronic inflammation.

- Liver Enzymes
  - o An imbalance of liver enzyme levels is associated with inflammation and cardio metabolic problems. The key enzymes are:

- ALT – Alanine aminotransferase
- AST – Aspartate Transaminase
- GGT – Gamma-Glutamyl Transpeptidase
- ALP – Alkaline Phosphatase

- Lipid Panel – HDL, LDL, Triglycerides
  - LDL:HDL ratio of 3:1 or less (2:1 is optimal)
  - Tri:HDL ratio of 2:1 or less (1:1 is optimal)
  - Higher rates may indicate insulin resistance and inflammation

- Vitamin D3
  - Low levels of vitamin D3 are associated with cardiovascular disease, inflammatory bowel disease, chronic kidney disease, non-alcoholic fatty liver disease and asthma.
  - These diseases are all highly linked to inflammation in the body.

APPENDIX TO CHAPTER 3

Adjusting to a Low-Carb Diet

When taking up a ketogenic diet or zero-carb diet, here are some pieces of advice that will help:

- There is a short adjustment period of a few days at the beginning of the diet. This is where your body's cells change-over from feeding on carbs to feeding on fats. For some people, it can feel pretty horrible, and you may need some serious mental stamina to get through it. Google "keto-flu" to find a lot of advice about making the transition period easier.

- Zero-carb is a whole other kettle of fish. Even if you have been eating a very low carb diet for some time, switching to zero-carb may involve another adjustment period at the start, in the same way that a ketogenic diet takes a few days of adjustment.

- It is vital that you increase your salt intake. You will definitely lose water weight on this diet, and salt will disappear with it.

- It will definitely help if you take electrolytes, such as magnesium, potassium, chloride. Most commercial electrolytes contain loads of sugar, but you can make an electrolyte drink yourself.

- Make sure you eat loads of fat, even if you already have lots of body fat. 75% of your calorie intake should be from fats. Failing to do this will make getting into ketosis very difficult, and can cause symptoms of starvation (eating up your muscles) and will prevent you from using your own body fat for energy.

- Watch out for hidden carbs. There are carbohydrates in everything - sauces, condiments, alternative milks, almost all packaged foods, etc. Common mistakes are eating tomato sauce, ketchup, salad dressings, especially the creamy ones like thousand island.

- When calculating protein levels in a food, remember that meat is not 100% protein. A beef steak weighing 100g may only contain 20g of protein. You can find the levels of protein, fat and carbohydrates in the food list provided in the Additional Information webpage for this book.

- Do not eat too much protein. This will bump you out of ketosis, and it will take some effort to start the process up again.

- Do not eat dairy. For many people this is pro-inflammatory, which can cause insulin resistance and prevent you from losing the weight you need to.

- Avoid commercial keto foods, and keto sweets. Look at this as keto junk food. For some people there are too many ingredients that cause inflammation, for others the zero-sugar sweets cause a rise in insulin as well as inflammation, along with cravings for more sweets. For many people, snacks are a temptation that leads them to exit the state of ketosis.

- Get more sleep. Ketosis can be stressful for the body at the beginning, and sleep will help. It will also help your efforts to reduce inflammation, insulin resistance and to lose weight.

Zero-Carb Diet Fats

- You need to know your fats – Butter, Ghee, Lard, Tallow, Duck Fat, etc. You might find that certain fats make you feel better than others. This can also change over time.

- Rendered fat (melted off the meat) often causes diarrhea. This is due to the change in structure of the fat when it is melted.

- And here are a few more tips that can help you succeed on this diet:

- Digestive issues are greatly improved on all-meat diets, and even better when those meats are cooked blue.

- It is best to start on a simple diet of steak, salt and water.

- Always buy meat that is fresh from a good butcher. Older meats, vacuum-sealed, from a supermarket or from a 2nd-rate butcher may cause problems.

- Do not eat anything that has been processed or aged, such as salami. These include extra ingredients (flour, milk products and sugar, believe it or not), and normally have loads of histamines.

- The same goes for hot dogs, sausages and even some bacon. These can include fillers, flour, sugars, bread crumbs, ketchup and possibly onion and other plants, plus a large dose of histamines.

- Aged steaks may be healthy, but also have extra high histamine content because of the aging. This may cause problems and it may be best to avoid any kind of meat that is not completely fresh.

- Mince, due to its larger surface area, can produce more histamine in a shorter time. If you like mince, you will need to make your own, or buy from a butcher that makes a fresh batch of mince every day. This precaution is not foolproof, since the grinding of the meat heats it up. Clever butchers actually throw the newly minced meat into the freezer for a while, to cool it down, to avoid problems.

- Don't cook with rendered fats at the beginning, like lard, tallow and even duck fat. These can cause problems for some people. Get used to the diet first, and then add some in later as a test. If you are frying, you don't need to use oils at all.

- If you are baking, keep the temperature between 100C and 150C to help keep prevent the fat from melting off the meat. This will also keep your oven and cooking area cleaner, because the fat doesn't pop and sizzle!

- Eat enough steak. One of the biggest problems people have is not eating enough. For a long time, I was eating one kilo of meat each day (including the fat)

- Make sure there is a lot of fat attached to the meat. This is where your energy supply comes from. If you cannot obtain meat with enough fat, add butter or ghee if you can.

- If you are eating out, there are hidden ingredients to be aware of:

  o Burgers almost always contain other ingredients, especially grain flours.

  o Scrambled eggs and omelettes often have batters added to create a fluffy texture.

  o Avoid toppings and sauces. Aside from sugars, these will contain a ton of flour for thickening, especially wheat, and often contain soy.

  o Marinades also are thickened with wheat, malt or soy sauce.

  o Imitation crab is primarily made from sugar, starches, egg, MSG and some kind of flavouring

  o Having Soup? Confirm that it is not made with vegetable stock, glutenous stock or bouillon. It needs to be a simple bone broth with no non-meat ingredients added.

This may seem like a large and confusing list, but take heart. It begins to make sense and becomes easy to remember over time. Also, the discussion in the nutrition section in book two explains a lot of the facts about plants, fats and intolerances in much more detail.

You may want to skip doing a keto diet and go straight to this style of eating. A zero-carb diet is also ketogenic and will improve your chances of eliminating reflux.

Further Tips:

Getting it right with testing ketones:

- Ketostix can be used at the beginning, to let you know you are starting to produce ketones. These are cheap, but they are not accurate, and are only an indication of ketone presence.

- Over time, ketostix will not pick up any ketones in the urine, because the body stops excreting them, as your body gets used to using them.

- For accurate results, invest in a small glucose/ketone meter. These can measure the amount of glucose, as well as the amount of ketones that you have in your blood system at any given time.

- Glucose/ketone meters are more expensive to use, but will give a good indication of whether you are getting the results that you are looking for.

APPENDIX TO CHAPTER 4

Medications that can cause reflux

- Pain Killers, NSAIDs such as Aspirin, ibuprofen, etc.

- Anticholinergics, such as oxybutynin (Ditropan XL), pre-scribed for overactive bladder and irritable bowel syndrome

- Tricyclic antidepressants (amitriptyline, doxepin, others)

- Calcium channel blockers, statins, angiotensin-converting enzyme (ACE) inhibitors and nitrates used for high blood pressure and heart disease

- Narcotics (opioids), such as codeine, and those containing hydrocodone and acetaminophen (Norco, Vicodin, others)

- Progesterone

- Sedatives or tranquilizers, including benzodiazepines such as diazepam (Valium) and temazepam (Restoril)

- Theophylline (Elixophyllin, Theochron)

APPENDIX TO CHAPTER 9

Here are the reasons why you need to raise your stomach acid. The chances are high that you know someone that suffers from one of these diseases, or maybe you recognize some of them in yourself. This is not an exhaustive list, of course! Although they can be caused by factors other than low stomach acid, low stomach acid often plays the pivotal role in the development of these diseases.

- Asthma in children
- Alcoholism
- Allergic Reactions
- Depression
- Rheumatoid Arthritis
- Chronic Autoimmune disorders
  - Lupus
  - Hypothyroidism
  - Hyperthyroidism
  - Gastritis
  - Celiac Disease

- Skin conditions including dermatitis, rosacea, psoriasis and eczema
- Flatulent dyspepsia
- Gallbladder disease
- Diabetes
- Osteoporosis
- Addison's Disease
- Anemia
- Ulcerative Colitis

- Gastric Polyps
- Myasthenia gravis (weakness of the muscles)
- Macular degeneration
- Multiple Sclerosis
- Osteoporosis
- Pernicious Anemia
- Scleroderma
- Sjogren's disease (dry eyes and mouth)
- Ulcerative Colitis
- Vitiligo
- Stomach Cancer

Methods to Diagnose Low Stomach Acid Levels

1. Baking soda test
2. Betaine HCL challenge test
3. Complete blood count CBC
4. Comprehensive metabolic panels CMP
5. Gastric acid secretion test
6. The Heidelberg stomach acid test

1. The baking soda test

This is the most precise and accurate test you can perform at home. For this, a person is asked to fast for at least 12 hours so that the stomach is devoid of food. Now dissolve a ¼ teaspoon of bicarbonate in a little amount of water and drink it on an empty stomach. The bicarbonate and stomach acid react chemically to produce carbon dioxide. The person performing the test should experience belching within five minutes of drinking the bicarbonate solution. If no belching occurs, it means the stomach acid levels are insufficient to react with bicarbonate and further testing should be performed by a doctor to determine the reason for the lack of stomach acid production.

2. Betaine HCL challenge test

This test is often provided as a test that can be performed at home, but I would advise against it. This test could indicate that you are producing enough HCl if you have a stomach condition such as atrophic gastritis. It may be better to take the baking soda test instead, if you are doing a home test.

However, here is an explanation about how this test is performed. To prepare for this test, eat a meal with plenty of protein content such as a steak (at least 30-40 grams of protein). Now, in the middle of the meal, take one capsule of Betaine HCl. Continue eating and monitor your symptoms. If you experience warmth in the stomach or chest area, it means your stomach acid levels are appropriate. If you feel nothing, this could be an indication of hypochlorhydria.

3. Complete blood count

A complete blood count is a medical test performed on a blood sample. The test gives the values of RBC, WBC, platelets, hemoglobin and hematocrit values in the blood. A low RBC count in the report indicates anemia, which is one of the potential signs of low stomach acid levels.

4. Comprehensive metabolic panel

Comprehensive metabolic panel is a diagnostic test that looks for the levels of metabolic components of body. The test gives the insight of

Iron levels

Iron requires stomach acid for its absorption in the body. Low iron levels in this test indicate hypochlorhydia.

Phosphorus levels

A low phosphorous test reading is an indication of low stomach acid levels, especially in conjunction with vitamin D deficiency.

Chloride levels

Chloride is an essential particle that makes up HCl. Therefore, the body requires a sufficient level of them for adequate HCl production. A low chloride ion test result indicates hypochlorhydia.

Blood urea nitrogen levels

A high blood urea nitrogen (BUN) reading is a sign that there is not enough stomach acid to remove nitrogen waste from the bloodstream. When the levels of stomach acid are low, the values of BUN rise sufficiently high to indicate hypochlorhydia.

Vitamin B12 levels

The blood analysis can provide an estimate of B12 levels. Low levels of this vitamin are a prominent marker of hypochlorhydia.

5. Gastric Acid secretion test

This test determines whether a person's stomach is capable of producing HCl. It is an invasive and costly test, so it is normally reserved for extreme cases. It requires the patient to fast for 4 to 6 hours so that the stomach is empty of food. Then a tube is inserted into the trachea to remove any existing gastric fluid. The hormone, gastrin, is then injected into the bloodstream, to stimulate the production of gastric acid. Any newly-produced acid is tested, and the pH values should sit at 1.5 to 3.5. If no acid, or very little acid, is produced after the injection of gastrin, hypochlorhydia is diagnosed.

6. The Heidelberg test

This test is the gold standard for stomach acid testing. It requires you to fast for 12 hours before the test. The test involves swallowing a small electronic device, about the size of capsule, whose function is to monitor pH levels in the stomach. After this you must drink a baking soda solution to neutralize any HCl in your stomach. From this point, the device records the amount of time it takes for the stomach to restore its proper level of acidity. If the level of stomach acid does not return to normal after the test, the person is said to have hypochlorhydria or achlorhydria.

SNEAK PEEK AT BOOK 2

What You Will Find in This Book

In this book, I concentrate on how food and nutrition affect us with acid reflux disease. Food tends to be the primary focus of most people that suffer from acid reflux, but as we saw in the first book, the way that we approach our food may have a greater impact on reflux than the food itself.

If you have not already read the first book, then this is not the place to begin. The first book in the series gives you the complete 'in a nutshell' explanation about how to overcome acid reflux. The first book, together with the accompanying recipes, could be all that you will ever need to achieve your goal.

This second book is for those that are looking for more in-depth explanations about the foods that we eat and how they may be affecting us. The world of nutrition is incredibly confusing, and the common lists of safe and harmful foods appear to be completely random and different for everyone. This is what we will be tackling here, to bring the foods we eat into groups that make sense.

This book cannot be read as some instruction, separate from book one. If the goal is to overcome acid reflux, then everything that is included here must be followed in the context of the low carbohydrate plans that were outlined in the first book. Remember that everything we discussed in the first book takes priority, and what we are discussing here is follow-on information that needs to be incorporated into the overall plan.

Is This Book for You?

And as I outlined in the introduction to Book 1, this book may not be for you if you are devoted to vegan and vegetarian meals. This series is all about what I found to be the quickest and most effective way to overcome acid reflux disease, from a personal perspective. In my own experience, tending toward vegetarian and vegan styles of eating did not help the situation, and the greatest improvements I have made have been with the inclusion of animal products.

Vegans and vegetarians may be able to overcome acid reflux using similar methods, but it would require the help of someone who is experienced in these eating styles so that the food components can be balanced to provide both healing and nutrition.

In fact, you will find that this book outlines some of the most important factors that I discovered about foods, and why I moved away from a plant-based diet. You will find out why many people have trouble with plant foods, and why some relief from a plant-based diet can bring relief from many different symptoms that originate from the digestive system.

The following chapters will investigate all the ways that plants can make the task of identifying 'trigger' foods an impossible task. You may be fine with a food one month, but react to it in the next. And some foods only react when eaten in combination, whereas alone they may be fine.

What you will find in the following chapters is not a list of trigger foods, or foods to avoid, but rather, what it is about a food that causes it to trigger your sensitivities. You will find that everything is categorized into classes and groupings of foods and their components, rather than a random cluster of do's and don'ts.

Have you ever wondered what the link is between all the 'trigger' foods that are listed on every website. Surely all those foods are not as random as they sound!

- Alcohol
- Fried Food
- Spicy Food
- Tomatoes
- Oranges
- Mint
- Beef
- Coffee
- Cheese
- Soda
- Chocolate
- Garlic & Onion
- Salt and Pepper
- Butter
- Candy

This is a very common list of reflux triggers, but in this book you will find them categorized into groups. The foods above can be grouped like this:

Group 1.   Alcohol, coffee, chocolate, candy, oranges, cheese, soda

Group 2.   Tomatoes and hot spices

Group 3.   Chocolate, pepper, spices

Group 4.   Oranges, chocolate, tomatoes, beef, cheese

Group 5.   Spicy food, pepper, chocolate, mint, coffee

Group 6.   Cheese, butter

You might notice that some of the foods here are listed in more than one group. This means that it has more chance of contributing to reflux disease. Chocolate, for example is listed here 4 times, making it more likely to be a problem. However, the good news is that once you understand how the food groups work, you may be able to arrange your life so that you can include any of these foods in your diet once again.

In fact, some of the foods listed as reflux triggers are actually completely safe in the right setting. There was a time that I couldn't eat beef or butter without reaction, but now I eat beef and butter almost exclusively. By the popular definition, I should be suffering reflux episodes all day long, but instead, it is this style of eating that has helped to eliminate the condition that I suffered with for so many years.

ONE MORE THING BEFORE YOU GO

It is impossible to contain everything inside one little book like this. I'm sure you will have a lot of questions, and I want to be able to provide you with the tools that will allow you to take care of your situation.

Please visit this site:

https://acidrefluxformula.com/book-1-additional-material/

This webpage has been created to accompany this book. It will be updated periodically to reflect information that you may need to know.

- Updates, additions or corrections that need to be made to this book in preparation for the next edition.

- Reference material to support the arguments in this book.

- Recipes to get you going on your journey.

- Lists of foods with their macronutrient levels (fat, protein and carbohydrate), so that you can calculate your own macronutrient consumption.

I would greatly appreciate it if you could leave a 5-star review for this book on Amazon. If you think this ebook and its accompanying material is worth less than 5 stars, please write to me and let me know what you think it is worth, as well as the information that you need to see to make it a 5-star product.

To provide this information, as well as any other opinions about this ebook, please feel free to write to me:

Book1@acidrefluxformula.com

I would love to hear any stories that you have about your situation and whether this information has been helpful for you.

I wish you well with your endeavors.

Sincerely,

Drew Niemeyer
Founder of *Acid Reflux Formula*

Printed in Great Britain
by Amazon